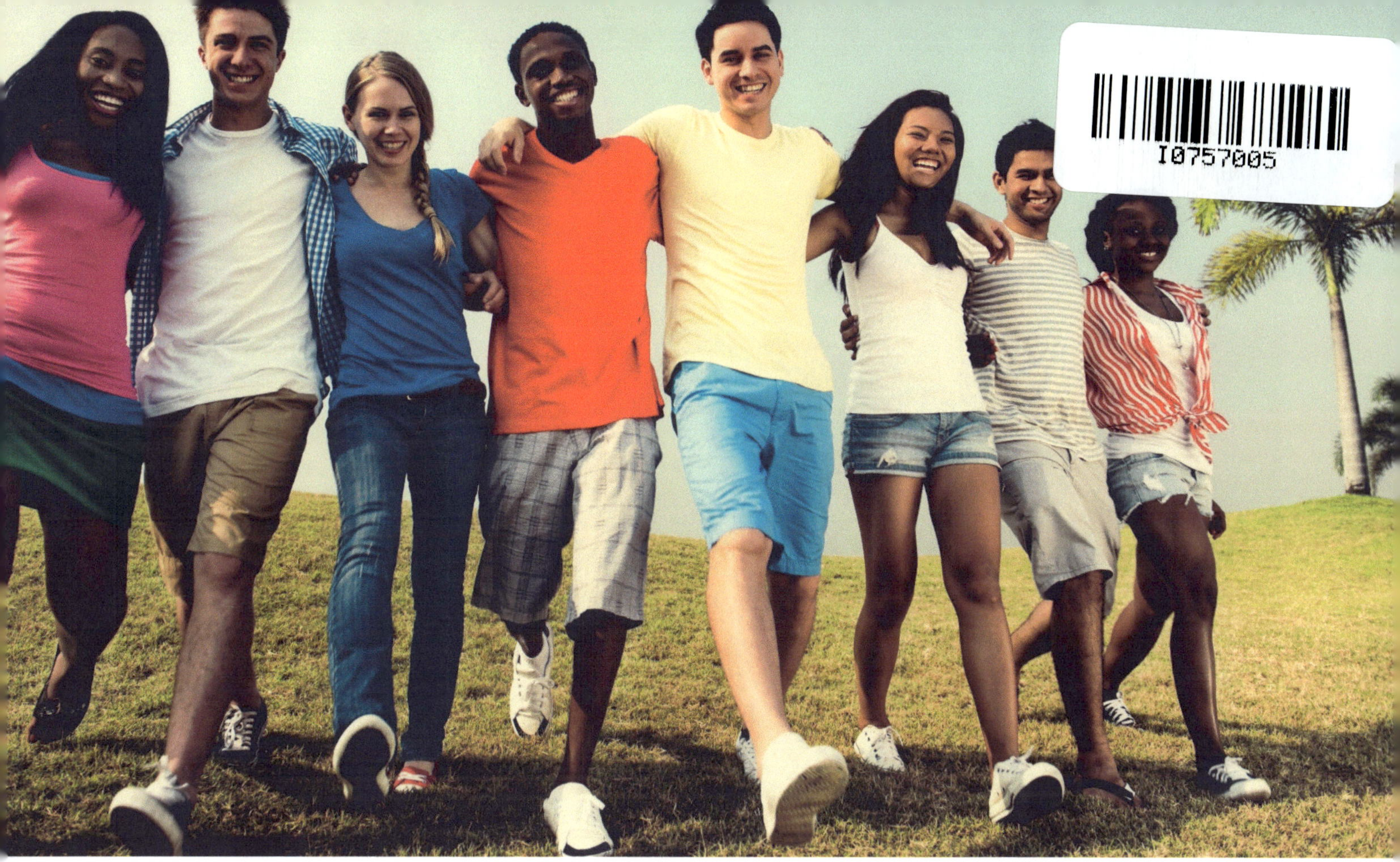

TOGETHERNESS

IT'S NOT HARD TO DO!

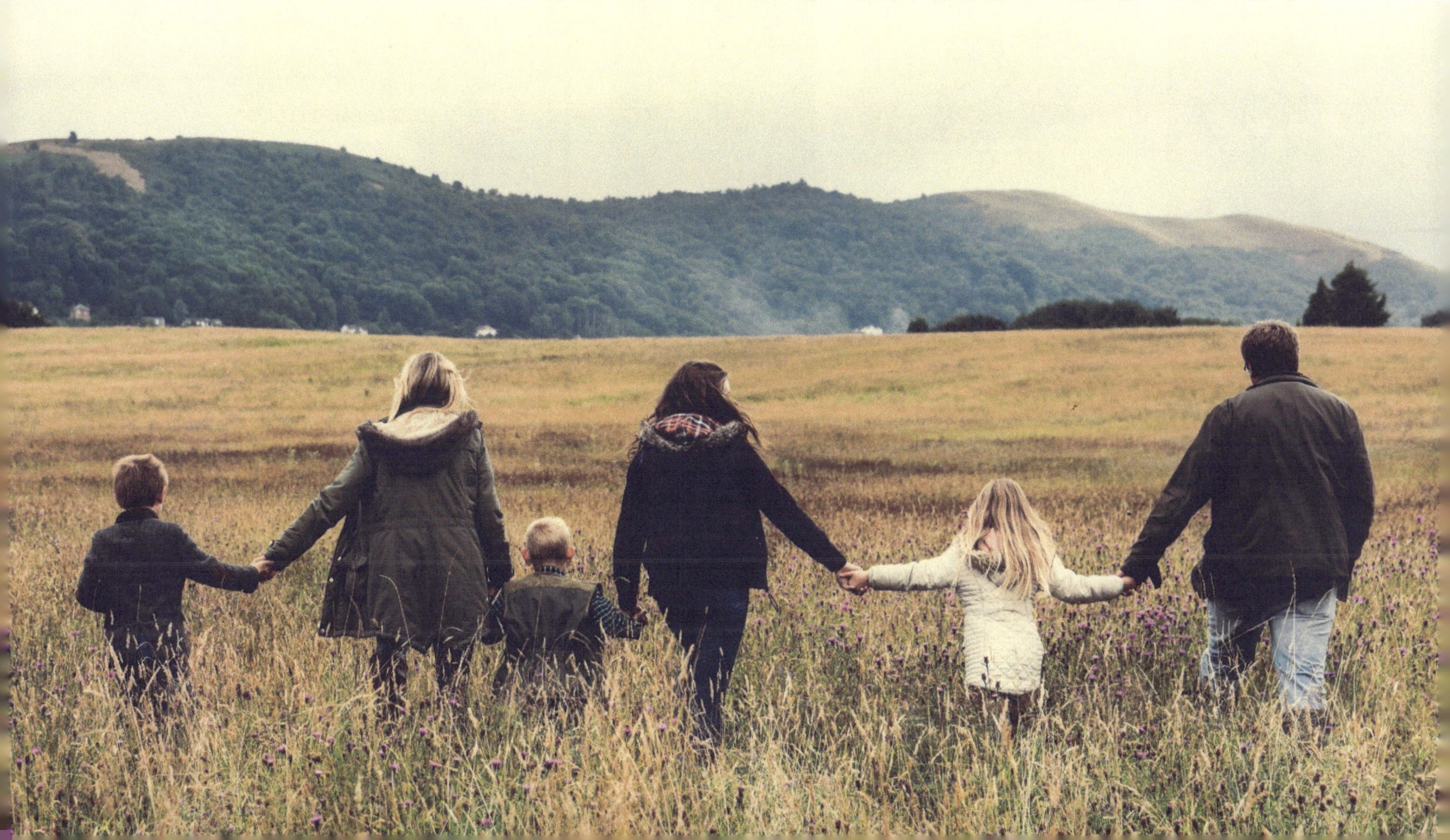

IMPACT ATLANTA MAGAZINE

Vanessa M. Henderson
Editor-In-Chief

Terri Stephenson
Managing Editor

Susan Jones
Founder/Layout/Publisher

Rod Murphy
Photographer

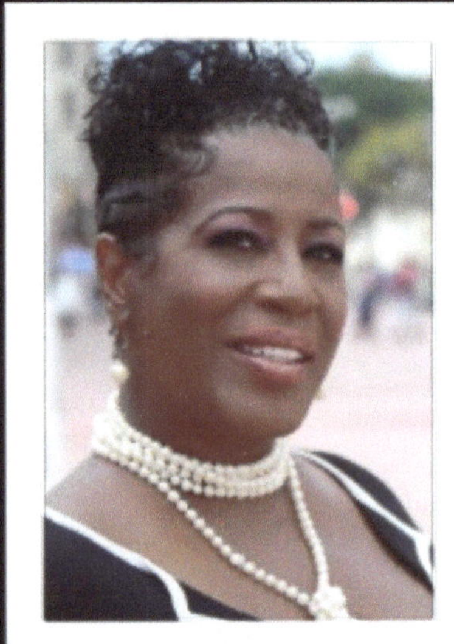

Terri Robinson-Stephenson
Managing Editor

A Letter from the Publisher

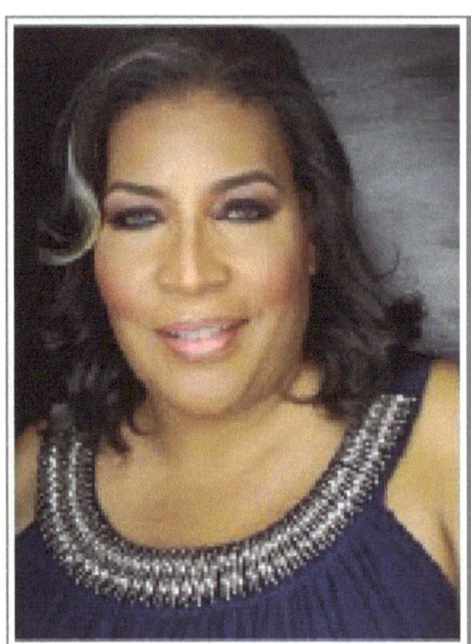

Susan Jones, Founder

Hello beautiful people. I'm Susan Jones, a publisher and innovator that prepares and issues books, magazines and other media. There are many great publishers, to which I acknowledge. However, what sets me apart is my drive and my diverse capabilities in all aspects of business, which allow me to produce content that resonates with people from all walks of life. I am a writer, a thinker, a friend, a business woman and also a baker.

At Impact Atlanta Magazine International, we find that often in the media the bad and the ugly consume the headlines in Atlanta and cities like her.

Sincerely,

~Susan Jones

Editoral

When we are focused.

Yes 2017 has come and gone. I can reflect on where we're going in the New Year. We see the trends of change. This has been a amazing year for Impact Atlanta International fashion and beauty.

We've had set ups and set backs ,but we moved through the world making strides. Moving to our first print issues in October. This was like Christmas for our team.

 We now realize that we have changed the game for you our readers forever. I invite you to continue to grow with us on this next level. Lastly know that in our world the sky isn't the limit. Feel the Impact.

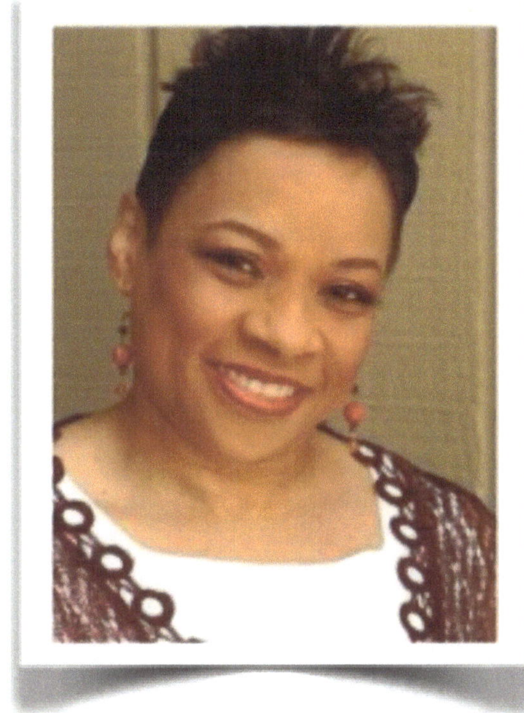

Editor-In-Chief
Vanessa M. Henderson
Editor-In-Chief

Contents

150 Quick &
Easy Recipes
to Transform
Your Body
Change Your Life By
Changing What You Eat

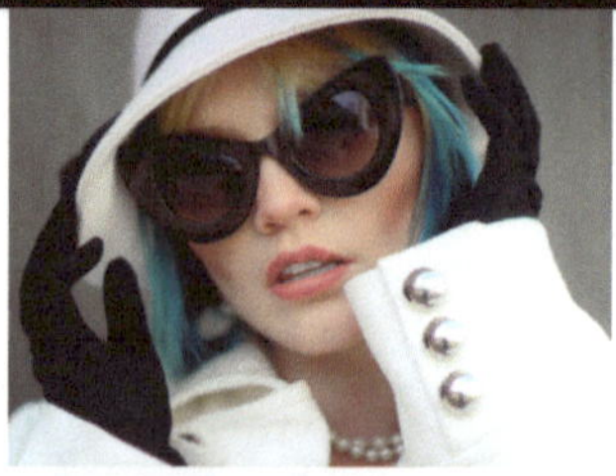

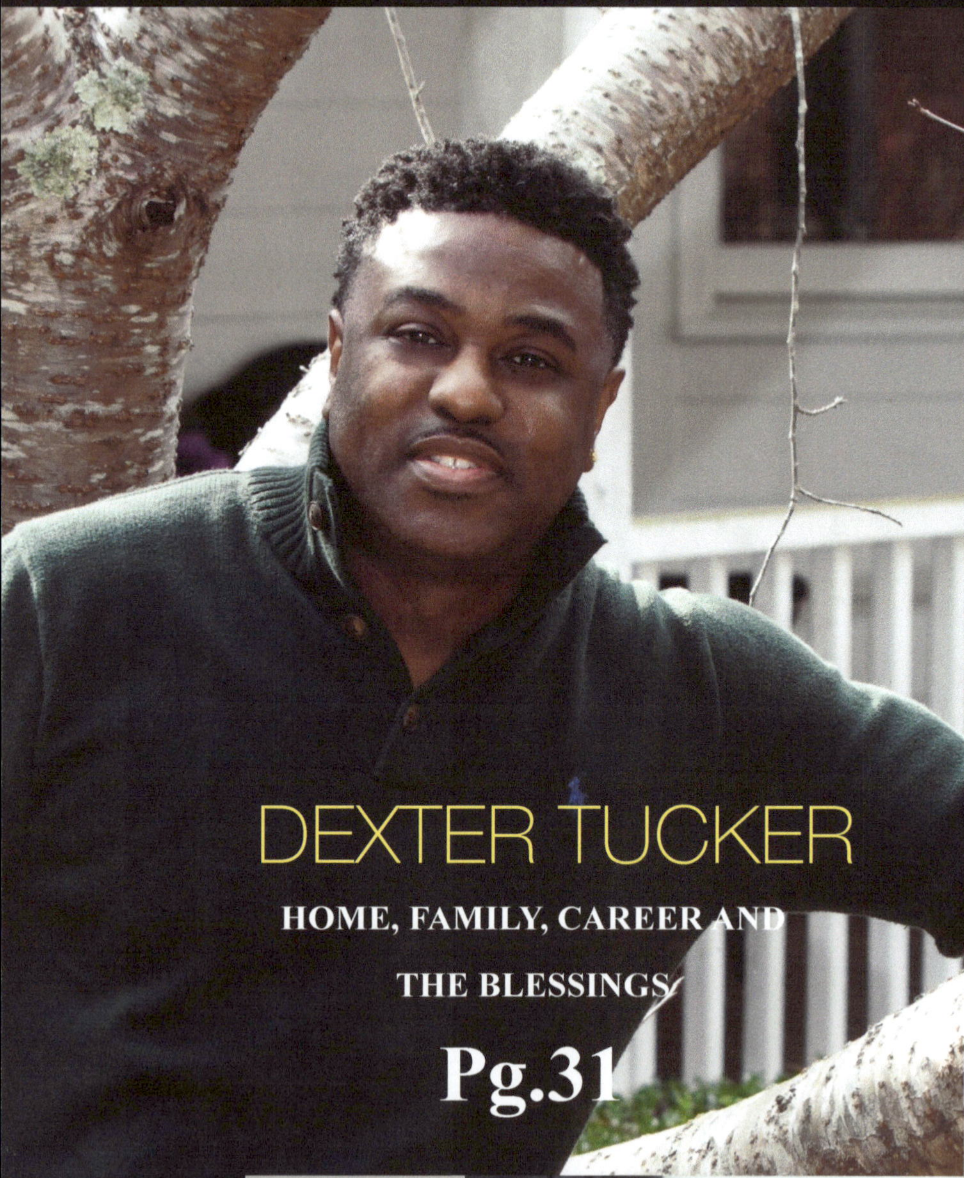

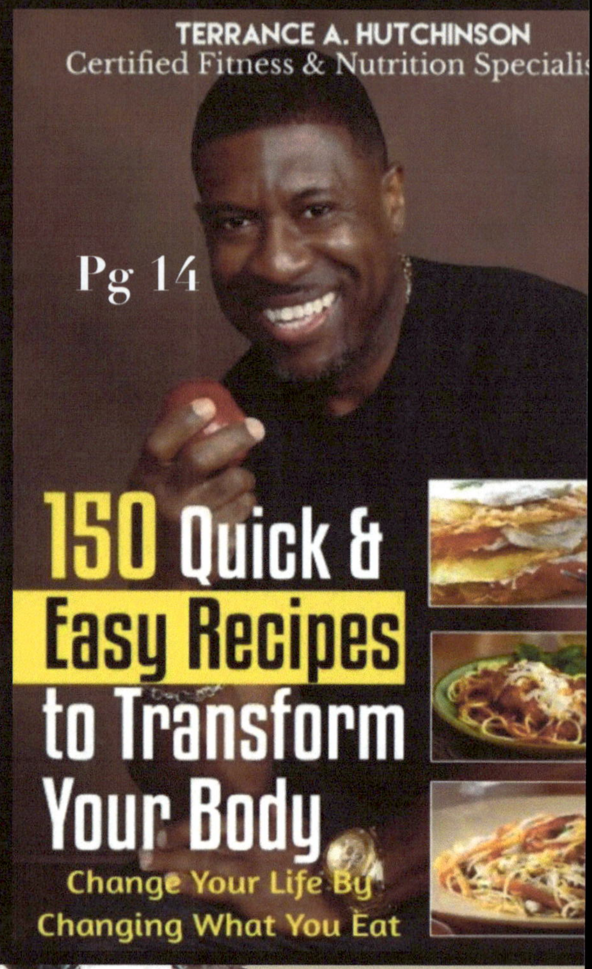

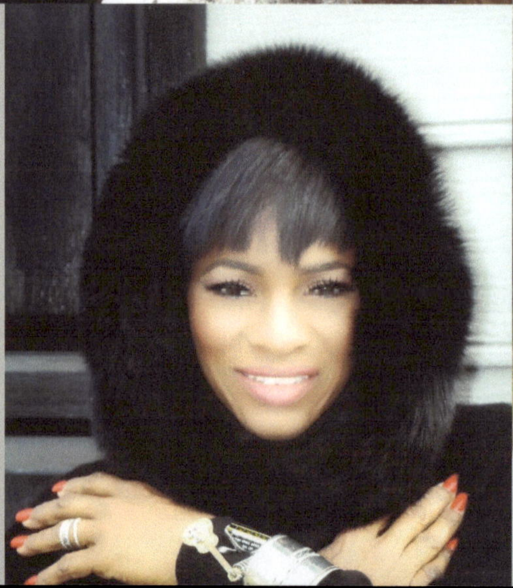

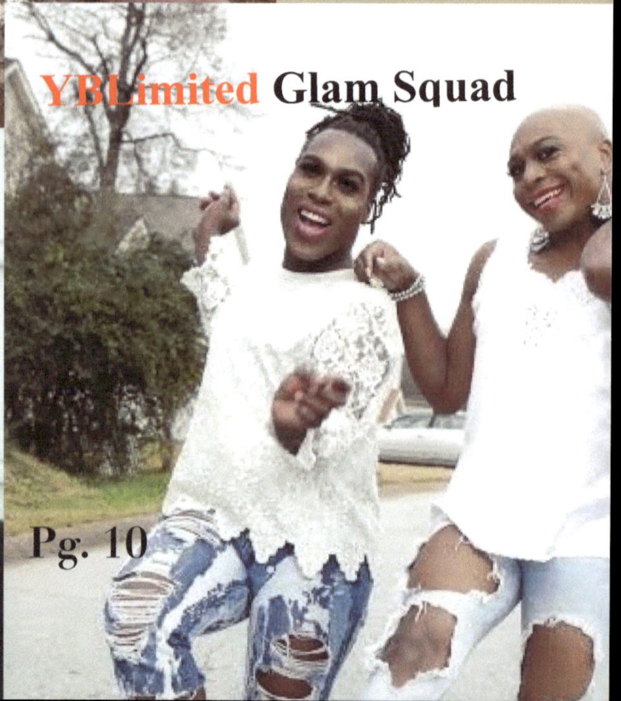

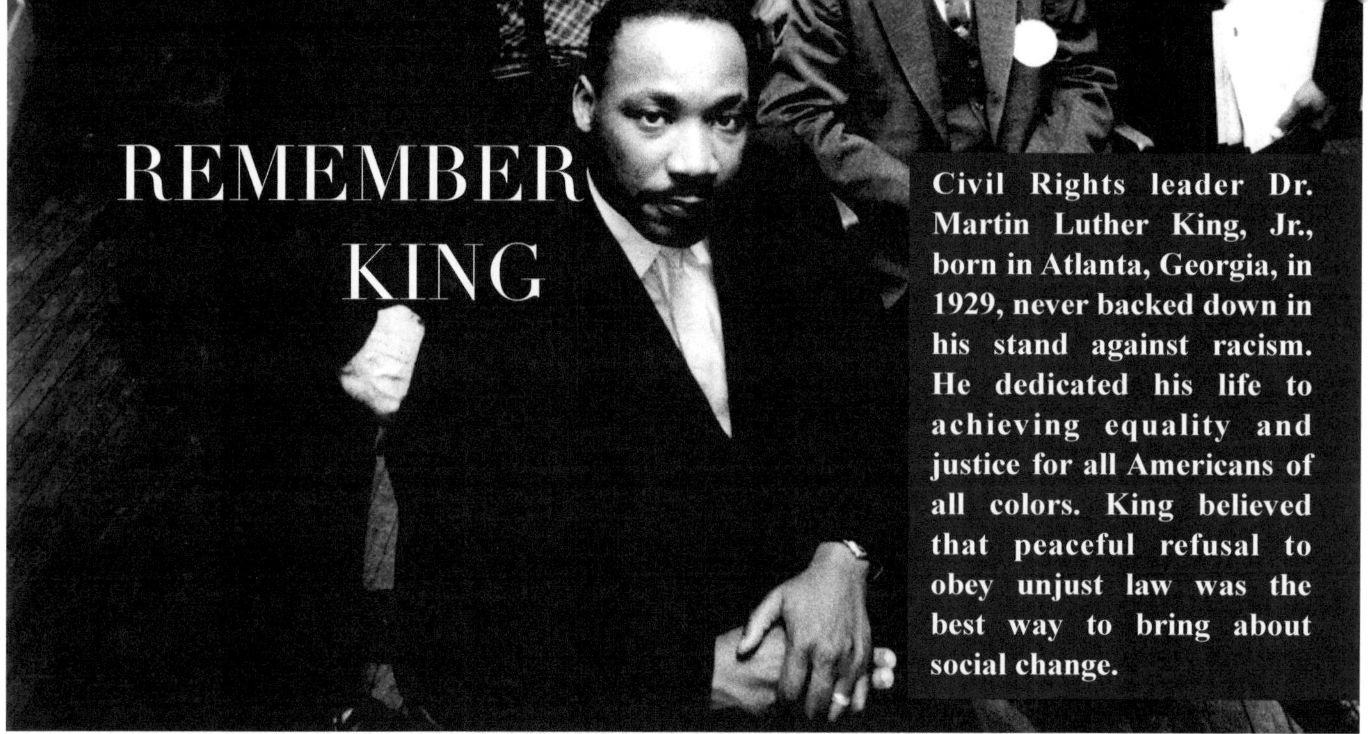

REMEMBER KING

Civil Rights leader Dr. Martin Luther King, Jr., born in Atlanta, Georgia, in 1929, never backed down in his stand against racism. He dedicated his life to achieving equality and justice for all Americans of all colors. King believed that peaceful refusal to obey unjust law was the best way to bring about social change.

Photograph by Donald Uhrbrock, Time & Life Pictures/Getty Images

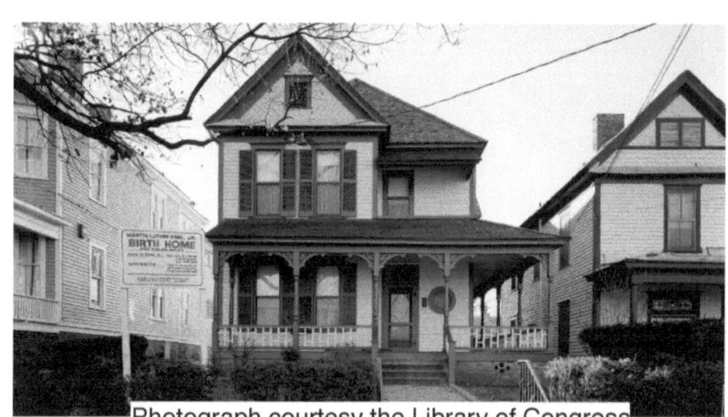

Photograph courtesy the Library of Congress

Dr. Martin Luther King, Jr.'s birth home still stands in Atlanta, Georgia. King experienced racial prejudice early in life. Segregation was both law and custom in the South and other

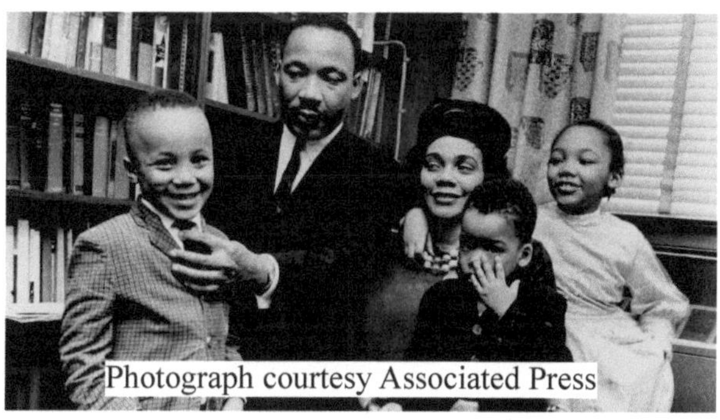

Photograph courtesy Associated Press

Dr. Martin Luther King, Jr. and his wife, Coretta Scott King, sit with three of their four children in their Atlanta, Georgia, home in 1963. His wife shared the same commitment to ending the racist system they had both grown up under.

Dr. Martin Luther King Jr waves to supporters from the steps of the Lincoln Memorial in Washington, D.C. during the "March on Washington." There, he delivered the "I Have a Dream" speech, which boosted public support for civil rights.

Photograph by AFP, Getty Images

A Few Good Men

by Duane Mollock

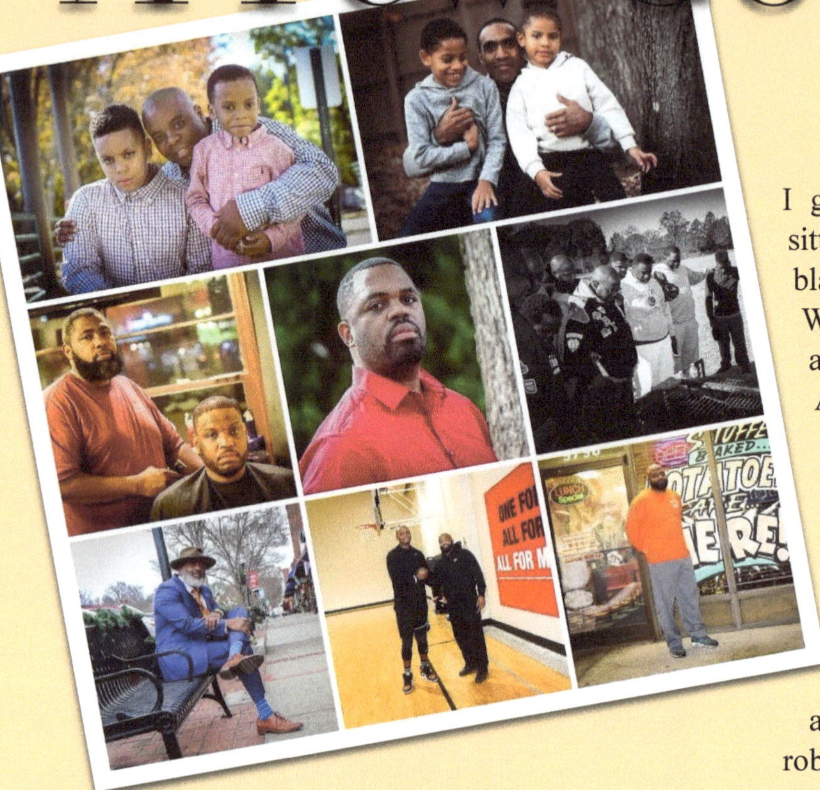

I got the idea for 'A Few Good Men' while sitting in the barbershop next to a 14-year-old black male, who was waiting on a haircut. While watching the evening news, segment after segment seemed to show African American males, ages 18-45, committing various crimes. It appeared as though no other race commits crime in America.

All of a sudden, the young man looked my way and asked a question.

"Sir" is that what the media think of us as a whole? Do they think we're all out here robbing, stealing and killing? " I immediately responded by saying, "No. The media focuses on the negative aspects of our community, and broadcasts that, as if it's the entire community."

In that moment, I decided to do something about it. I decided to use my camera as a weapon to combat the mass volume of negative images portrayed in the media of African American males.

Incredible...What kind of impact or benefit do you think a project like this will have on kids?
I think a project like this can have a tremendous impact on our youth, simply because most kids wants to become an athlete or entertainer. Unfortunately, everyone can't make it as a professional athlete or entertainer. The odds that it takes to become successful as a pro athlete or entertainer are a million to one. I believe this project will shed light on what other forms of success looks like for our youth. There's an old saying, "When we shift our perception, our experiences change." With that

How did you get your start?

In my youth (during the 90's,) I used to produce records for several major labels. Consequently, several of those records went on to sell huge numbers. I wrote, produced and remixed various artists' material, such as Montell Jordan, Coolio, Portrait, E40 and Ahmad's hit single, "Back In The Days," which was featured in the movie, "The Wood." Ironically, the movie took place in Inglewood, California, which happens to be where I was raised during my adolescence. In total, I produced/wrote over 33 songs that sold in excess of 3.5 millions records worldwide.

Unfortunately, you're only as big as your last hit record. So, I had to start over. I ventured into corporate America as a sales and business development consultant. It's a career that I like, however, the creative bug never left. That's what lead to my interest in photography.

What inspired you to create such a positive artistic expression?

being said, when you look at other cultures such as the Asian communities, whether they are Chinese, Japanese or Korean, the perception is that they are smart people. But the reality is, all of a hundred years ago, that wasn't the case. Not saying it wasn't true, but the point is that wasn't the general perception in American Society. But they did something about it. They took control of the way people perceived their culture, supervised the narrative of images portrayed in the media, which now projects that they're highly intelligent. Therefore, they no longer receive second-class treatment. And I think the same thing can be applied in the African American community.

Absolutely, Let's shift that perspective to adult women. By seeing this project not only from the context of your lens, but perhaps seeing up close in their community, hopefully more often than not, what kind impact do you think it will have on females in the community?

In terms of the impact the project will have on females in our community, I think the more images they see of everyday black men getting married, raising families, keeping a steady source of income, Black men that are actively striving to do something positive in their community, I believe that would give them a sense of respect for their male counterparts and potential mates. If everybody around you is thinking the same, it's easy to fall in that trap.

The goal was to capture different walks of life, with brothers doing different things, whether they're dealing with their families, running a business, or working with at-risk teens. Contrary to popular belief, these are the UNSUNG heroes that we see every day that never receive publicity. I've seen them all my life. From my Grandfather, Uncles, Neighbors and mentors.

Wow.... Last, but not least, let's talk about the impact your project will have on other men or friends and friends in the community. How do you think your project will impact on all of those levels?

Well, I think we live in the microwave age where everybody wants success and monetary gain instantaneously. I think the men involved with this project, are a clear example of black men who has the same amount hours per day, per week, per year, that chose to do something productive with their time. The one thing they all have in common is they try to improve themselves by 1% per day. If you think about it that is a 365% improvement year over year.
In addition, each subject shares a principle or rules that they live by, which I think can help others in the future. But internally your power comes from within. You're already rich if you have your health and good relationships with people. But, ultimately, it is up to you to do something with it.

With that being said, you have already set the foundation. This project will be a success not only with your vision and passion but with people who jumped on board and joined your movement. Congratulations.

I also want to add one thing. If you think about it, in the 50's and 60's, neighborhoods like Harlem, Central Avenue in Los Angeles, or any other predominantly black neighborhood, those areas were considered proud communities. If you look at your grandparents old photo albums, that's what you would see. They didn't have a lot, but they had a lot because they were proud of themselves and they projected that image, and that was the perception of us. There was a time when major corporations marketed to the black consumer because you had two parent homes with discretionary income. Again, people didn't have a lot, but they were very proud people.
A few years ago, The ALS Challenge went viral. So, I challenge the community to make this go viral. How the seed of 'A Few Good Men' could impact how the world perceives us, by us conducting ourselves in a positive manner.

HOW TO AVOID COLD WEATHER WOES

(BPT) - As sweater season knocks on the door, it's time to prepare for the brisk temperatures ahead. This winter, keep your home, health and well-being top of mind with these simple tips to avoid cold weather woes.

Winterize your porch

Install plexiglass panels to keep the cold weather out, allowing you to host friends and family, protect your furniture from snowfall and minimize spring cleaning. Once winter is over, simply pack up the panels and store

drips or pooling. For added convenience, connect the device to your cell phone to receive alerts in real time.

Turn it upside down

To warm your home without drastically increasing the gas bill, simply reverse the ceiling fan direction. During the summer months, ceiling fans push air down, naturally lending a cooling effect to those below. By reversing the ceiling fan upward, the cooler air is redirected, keeping you and your family

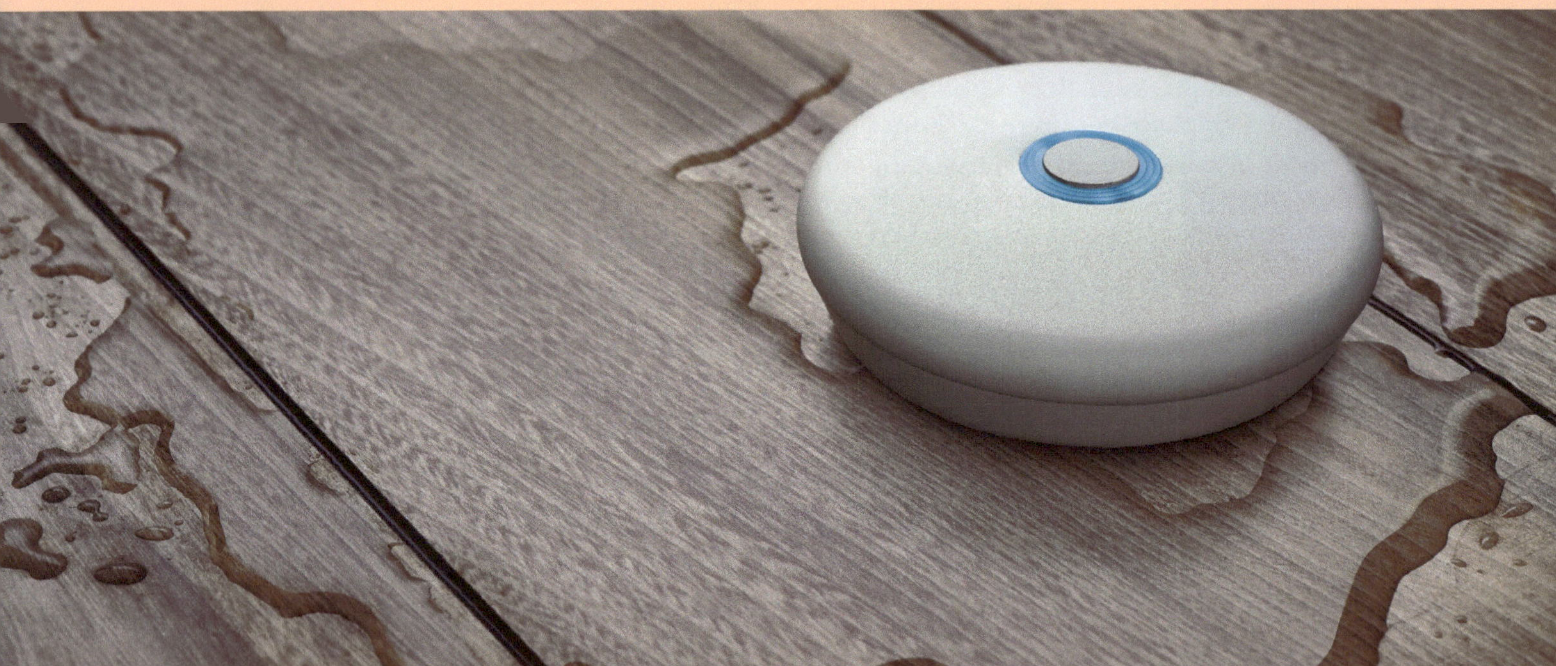

them for next season. For those who splurged on flooring, apply a protective finish, such as a water sealer or stain, to ensure excess moisture does not seep through the wood.

Take preventative measures

Oftentimes, frozen pipes can burst throughout the winter, or cause leaks as they begin to thaw in the spring. Keep your home safe from leaks by installing the Delta Water Leak Detector — a device that identifies leaks quickly and alerts homeowners at the onset. Simply place the leak detector near water heaters, appliances, sinks or toilets to detect

warm beneath.

Cozy up your home

To battle dreary days, stock up on warm essentials, such as flannel bedding, down throw blankets and plush towels. Outfit the common areas with warm fabrics and decorative patterns to keep your home cozy and welcoming during the winter. Finally, consider purchasing comfortable rugs and mats to keep your toes warm on tile and wood floors.

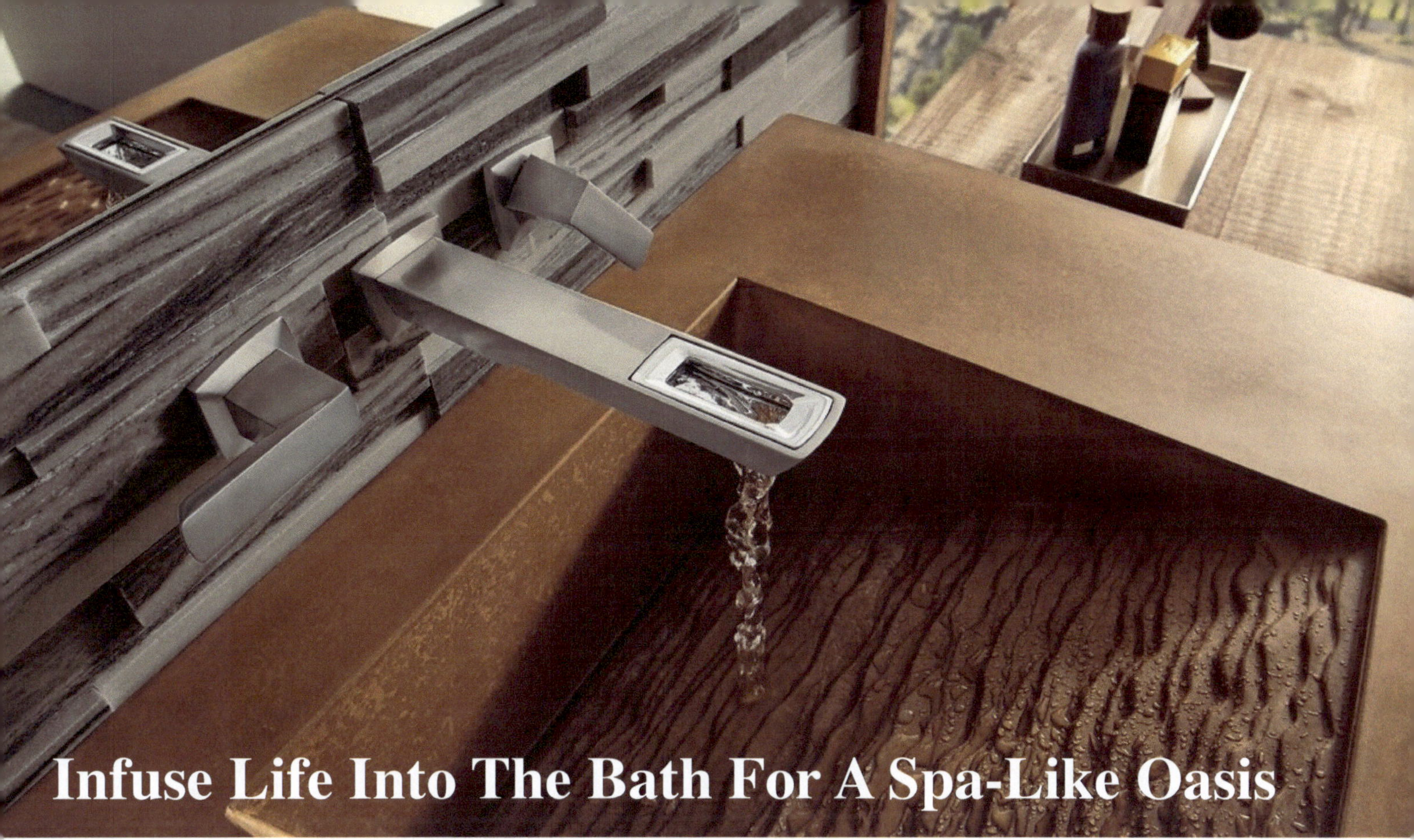

Infuse Life Into The Bath For A Spa-Like Oasis

(BPT) - Today, more than ever, homeowners gravitate toward design elements that transform the bath into a spa-like oasis. Designers look to incorporate pieces inspired by the natural world to bring renewed energy into the room and create a soothing environment. From fixtures inspired by booming waterfalls, to neutral color schemes and natural light, nature infuses life back into luxury bath design for a serene sense of calm.

Neutral Calm

Light colors such as cool grays and muted blues evoke tranquility and peacefulness. Neutral colors for walls and fabrics create a soothing aesthetic that fosters relaxation in the space. To create visual interest within a neutral palette, incorporate varying shades of earth tones to serve as complementary accents throughout the room — from decorative rugs and plush towels to cabinetry and tiling.

Nature's inspiration

Elements inspired by nature work together to produce a sense of relaxation in the home's oasis. Intuitive in design, the Vettis Bath Collection by Brizo combines solid proportions and angular architecture with an optional four-sided open chamber that mimics the sensory experience of a waterfall. Inspired by the strength found in nature, the defined edges of the spout create a balanced aesthetic, while subtle facets offer visual depth. Paired with natural stone accents, this collection evokes elements of natural inspiration.

Stone serenity

A freestanding stone tub makes a luxurious statement to enhance the spa atmosphere. Sleek, oval architectures provide an organic contemporary touch, while rectangular basins deliver a strong geometric focal point. Take the spa-like experience even further and incorporate the use of essential oils. Lavender and chamomile reduce stress and encourage sleep, while peppermint and lemon oils increase focus and mental alertness in the morning. From modern to transitional aesthetics, a freestanding, natural stone tub paired with the sensory infusion of essential oils creates the perfect at-home getaway.

Living accents

Natural lighting and live plants blur the line between the great outdoors and the enclosed space. Large floor-to-ceiling windows and skylights serve as eye-catching accents while also naturally illuminating the room. Hanging succulents and potted bamboo plants are additional decor options to bring nature indoors without sacrificing clean, simple design.

YBL United
Glam Squad

Story / Make-up / Wardrobe by Phillip Washington & Henrico St. Fleur

Photo: Wayne Bagley

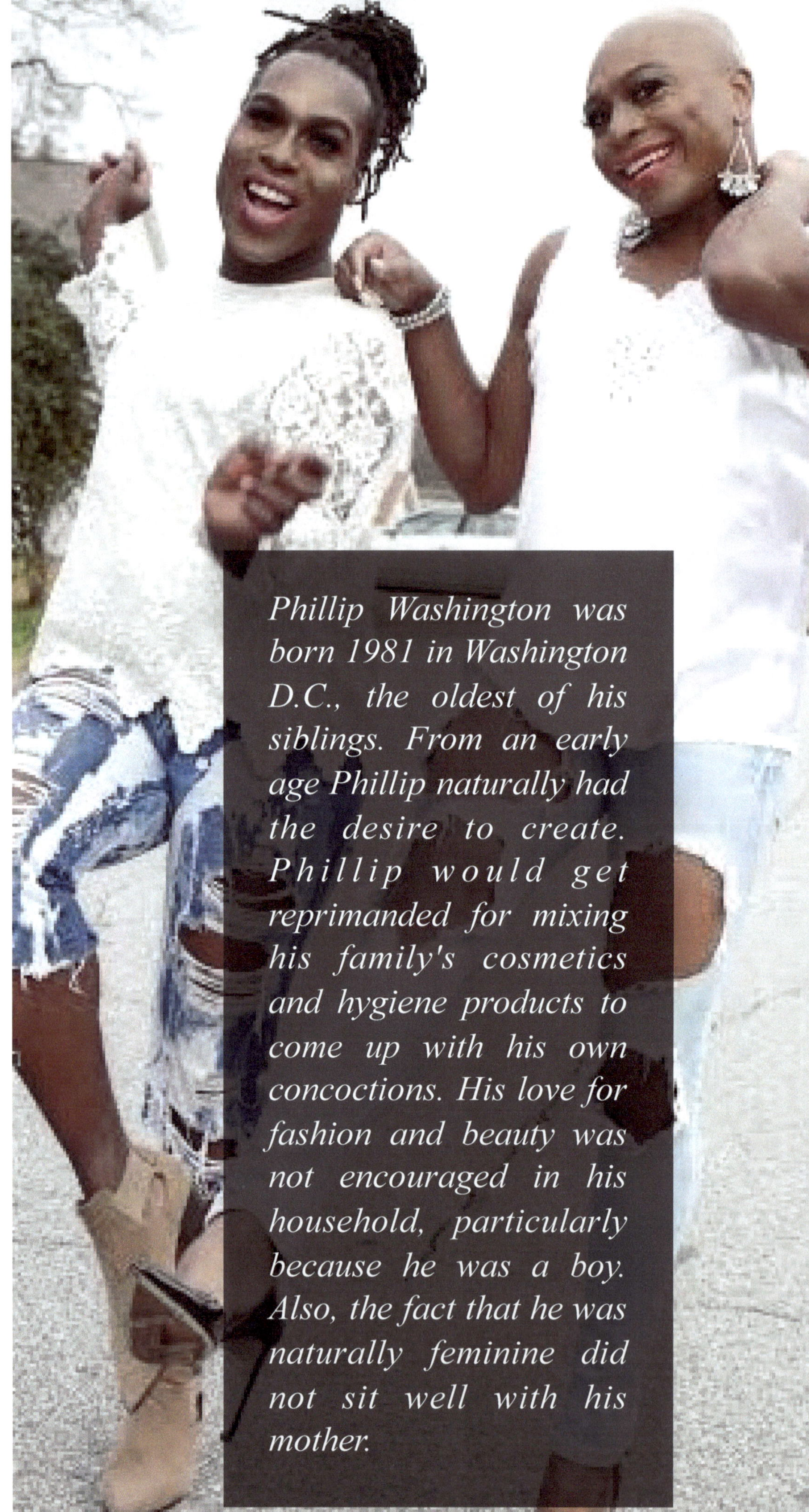
Phillip Washington was born 1981 in Washington D.C., the oldest of his siblings. From an early age Phillip naturally had the desire to create. Phillip would get reprimanded for mixing his family's cosmetics and hygiene products to come up with his own concoctions. His love for fashion and beauty was not encouraged in his household, particularly because he was a boy. Also, the fact that he was naturally feminine did not sit well with his mother.

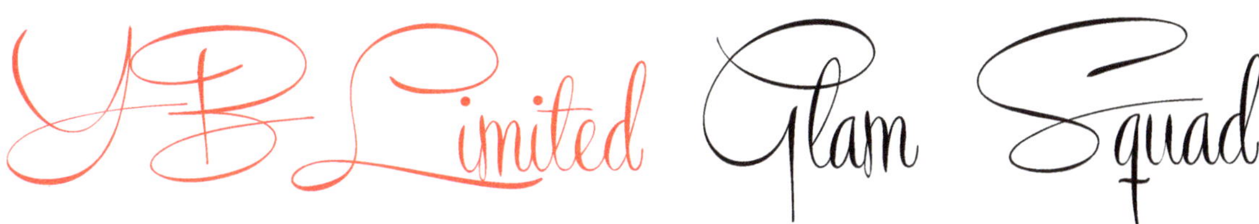

Phillip began to secretly steal his cousin's Barbie dolls to do their hair because he felt his cousin was not doing Barbie any justice. Every time his mother would discover a hidden doll he would be disciplined. Slowly Phillip withdrew from embracing his love for beauty in order to avoid the consequences and ridicule he would experience from home. Instead he replaced his love for fashion and beauty with trying to fit in with the "in crowd." Slowly he lost in individuality and forgot how much he loved the world of art and creation. Little did he know that trying to

"fit in" was gradually breaking him down. Phillip then turned to drugs to cope with the pain of feeling different from mainstream society. After losing his job at a flourishing entertainment management company, Phillip's personal and professional life fell faster than anyone could ever imagine. Phillip became homeless due to his addiction. Along with numerous near death overdoses. After spending two years in prison and beginning the journey of self-discovery, Phillip's life never looked the same.

Meanwhile unbeknownst to Phillip, in 1986 down in Miami, FL, Henrico St. Fleur was born the third of four children. Henrico comes from a Haitian background where life was a hard living. As a charismatic and very artistic young boy, he was also often misunderstood. Henrico's energy was considered too much for the other children. All he wanted was to fit into a society. Instead society kept reminding him that he was "wrong." As a child, Henrico (Rico for short) always found himself looking

out the window and on the other side was a world he was afraid to experience. It all changed for him when he realized that he did not have to stay on that side of the window. Henrico had the power to walk out there and create a world as he saw it. A world he wanted to explore. The rejection from society motivated him to create a world that was safe and all inclusive. From there he started telling his story through a lens. A friend of his would always asked him, "Rico, what makes you?" Henrico's replay? "Honey, My NAME silly." He knew his name "Henrico" was destined for greatness. As he lived and allowed life to

Both of the young men were homeless and in two different transitional centers. Shortly after they met they became one another's strongest supporters.

present itself, Henrico finally realized he was incorrect about what made him. Today he can honestly say what makes him is his life experiences. Which has not always been a piece of cake. For as long he could remember he was fascinated by smells, moods, feelings, habits, and the activities of life. The awareness of these things created his love for photography and its seven elements (in no particular order), texture, line, color, shape, form, tone and space. This was done by capturing others' lives through the art of photography. Henrico would go to school with six disposable cameras. He would be so excited to take them to the one hour photo to get developed. Since he did not have any money, he would pick out the ones he loved and kept it moving, without paying. After months of returning to the one hour photo store they finally caught on to what was going on. Needless to say he wore out his welcome.

Henrico found an outlet in the world he created with photography, still the rejection of childhood would often haunt him. Henrico would find himself making a series of poor choices that in his early adulthood left him homeless and in trouble with the law. At times he would neglect his safe place called photography to focus more on the streets that falsely appeared to accept him. Then in the mid-2000s, Henrico made a choice to come to Atlanta. No one knew that this particular choice would change, and maybe save, his life. It was not until a few years after moving to Atlanta that he made a conscious decision to turn his life around. Shortly after making that decision, at a support group, Henrico ran into Phillip Washington who was recently released from prison.

Both of the young men were homeless and in two different transitional centers. Shortly after they met they became one another's strongest supporters. They became roommates and naturally began to create. Everywhere Henrico and Phillip would go would become a photo shoot, and a major production. They would create high end photos, with a flip phone. It was in the 90s when Henrico got his first start as a photographer using a disposable camera. So the flip phone was considered an upgrade. Although Henrico did end up working at photography studios in his late teens, it was his early experience with a disposable camera that he taught himself the difference from "the photographer" and "the photograph." One creates, and the other express what has been created. That rule goes for any artist. Today, he doesn't just take pictures of the crowds. Henrico focuses on a small portion to convey God at its best, and in its likeness.

At this point Phillip had become known for the homemade lip gloss he created himself while in prison. People would tell Phillip and Henrico that they should start a lip gloss line. At first they thought it was a bit farfetched to become entrepreneurs. Except both Phillip and Henrico had learned through their journey of self-discovery in their personal lives that they could do ANYTHING they wanted, regardless of their background. After encouragement from their friends, they sat down to start a company together. Even though it was originally supposed to be a lip gloss company, they know that God did not have limits and that they did not know what plans God had for their new company in the future. After making a couple of pages with names that looked too limited they asked themselves, "Why-b Limited?" That is when the light bulb went off for them both. They knew that they did not know where God would take their brand, so they affectionately distorted the spelling to form what is now known as "YBLimited."

From the very beginning the company took on its own life. It started with Phillip simply making his own version of luxury lip gloss from scratch, and he quickly transitioned into a self-taught makeup artist. Henrico would come to photograph Phillip's work so that his work and the company would be shown in the most professional light. That is what prompted them to create YBLimited Mobile Glam Squad in 2013. YBLimited was the first and only all-inclusive mobile services company in the country. They recruited some of the top beauty and fashion professionals to be a part of YBLimited. They ended up with over a dozen accomplished hairstylists, makeup artists, photographers, and wardrobe stylists. After doing makeup and photography for the producers of the BET Awards in 2014, the celebrities and television shows came calling for YBLimited Mobile Glam Squad. The YBLimited Glam Squad started to be in high demand around the country. YBLimited managed to make over twenty national publications in a little over a year. After helping numerous professional actors and models build their portfolios, YBLimited naturally evolved into forming the model management division of YBLimited in mid-2017.They took on three professional models/actors to both manage through YBL Model Management, and to also utilize them as YBL brand ambassadors. The latest venture for Phillip and Henrico has taken them full circle to FINALLY launching the lip gloss collection they originally began with four years ago under the YBLimited umbrella. This journey has shown both Phillip and Henrico that the power of art and creativity has no limits, and neither do they. That is why in everything they do they set out to create an experience that will cause whomever they encounter to ask themselves, "YB-limited?"

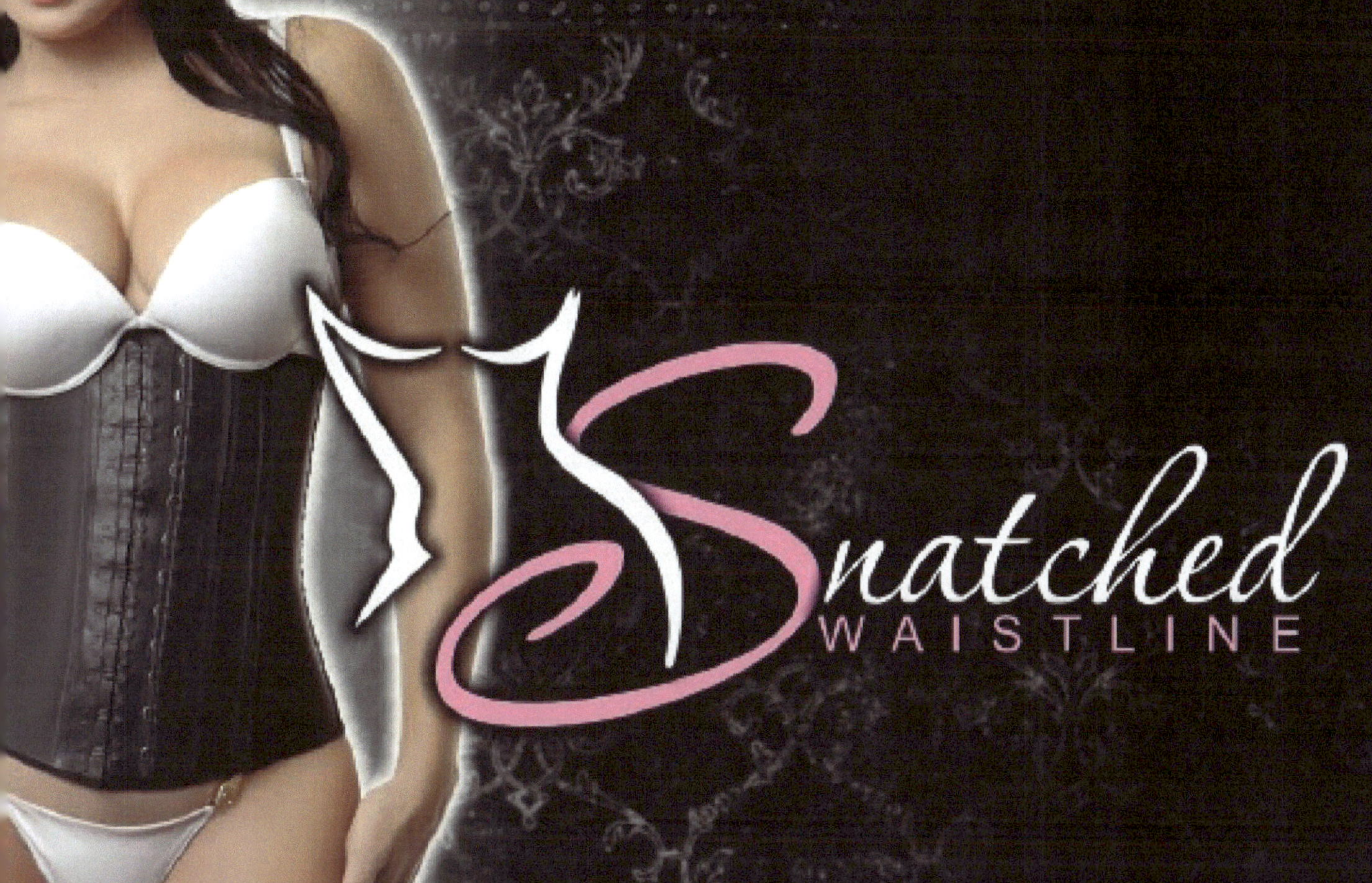

Waist Trainers Starting at $40.00

470-535-2528

TERRANCE A. HUTCHINSON
Certified Fitness & Nutrition Specialist

150 Quick & Easy Recipes to Transform Your Body

Change Your Life By Changing What You Eat

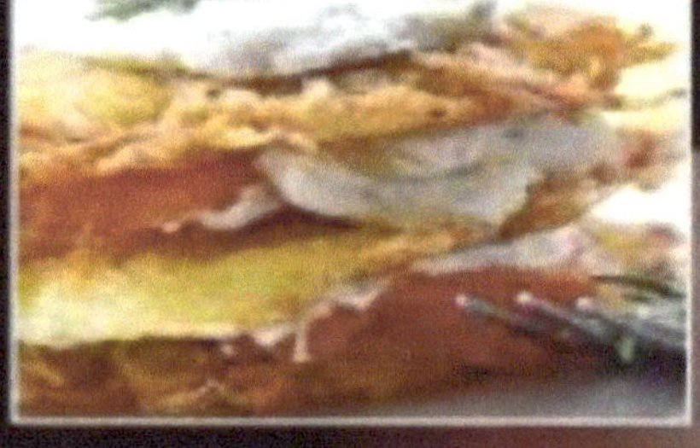

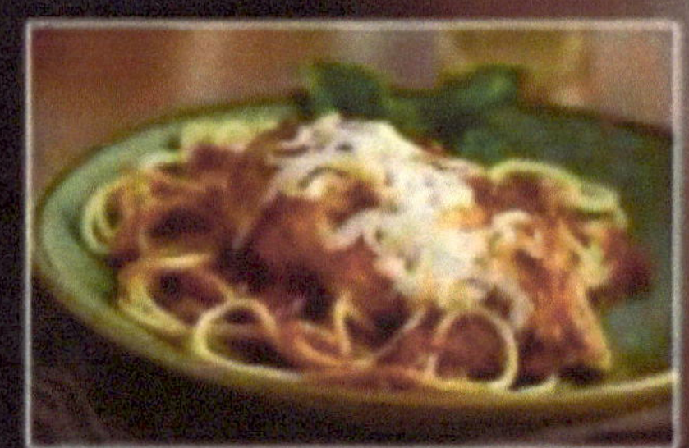

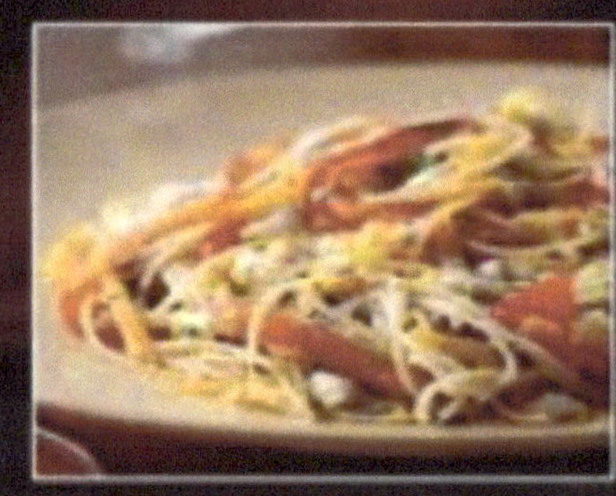

Best Lifestyle Fitness and Nutrition

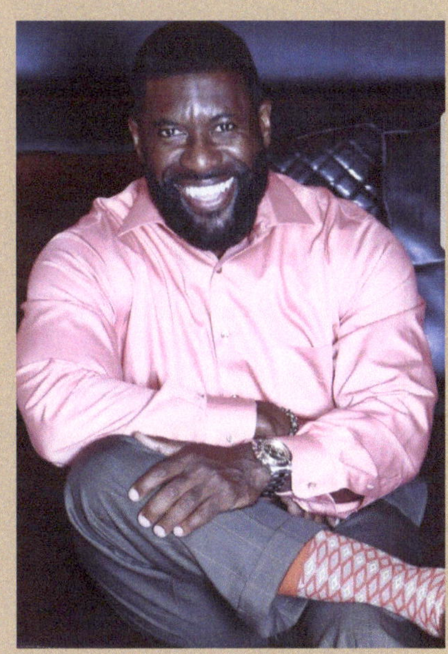

Who is Terrance Hutchinson and how do you stand out from the rest?

Who is Terrance Hutchinson ? Well, Terrance Hutchinson is the owner of *Best Lifestyle Fitness and Nutrition.* I have been providing health and fitness instruction over the last 9 years throughout Georgia, Carolinas, Florida, and New York areas. We also have online fitness programs with clients in Germany and Australia.

I am a Certified Fitness and Nutrition Specialist, Certified Corporate Consultant, Certified Exercise Therapist, and the author of 150 Recipes to transform your body and 25 irresistible Dessert that you can Indulge in Cook Books. Terrance is the host of *The Total Wellness Show* with Terrance on WBQE Blazin

Radio 95.2, and motivational speaker.

What are some of your accomplishments?

I have been nominated for the 2017 *Rice Awards* for health and wellness, Atlanta Hottest author, fitness model, an online radio host. Nominated for best self magazine's best personal trainer in Atlanta for 2017. Also, a cover model for *Bold Ageless Beauty Magazine's* fall issue; also was nominated for *Bold Favor Magazine's* for Health and Wellness.

My company is currently in partnership negotiations with local Physical Therapist and Chiropractors to help bring their patients to a more well round recovery experience.

I have coached dozens of people in their homes, fitness centers, corporate offices, boot camps, nutritional guidance seminars, HIIT circuits, Power Training, and in-home Personal Chef, with demonstrations into successfully leading others to a healthier lifestyle.

Furthermore, I am a lead in-services, consultations and diabetic classes to local hospitals, Corporate Wellness programs around the Atlanta area on exercise fundamentals and proper nutrition for a healthier lifestyle makeover.

What are some of the things that you do to put forth your platform?

I'm a active advocate for promoting disease prevention, promoting proper nutrition, purposeful physical exercising, and corporate wellness strategies in the work place.

I'm always continuing my education and putting into practice the newest leading edge techniques to ensure true results! Terrance's goal is to shape and influence the health and fitness attitudes of those around him and Best Lifestyle Fitness and Nutrition to make the dream of optimal health a reality.

At this stage in your life how do you create a work and life balance?

I understand how it is to maintain a busy work schedule while balancing proper nutrition and purposeful exercise. Whether it's to lose or gain weight, increase strength, continue post rehabilitation after prescriptive medical care or creating customized programs for clients, I have expertise in all areas of the fitness and wellness industry. I truly believe that with education, diligence, dedication, commitment, and the motivational coaching, everyone can live the dream of achieving the body and health of their dreams.

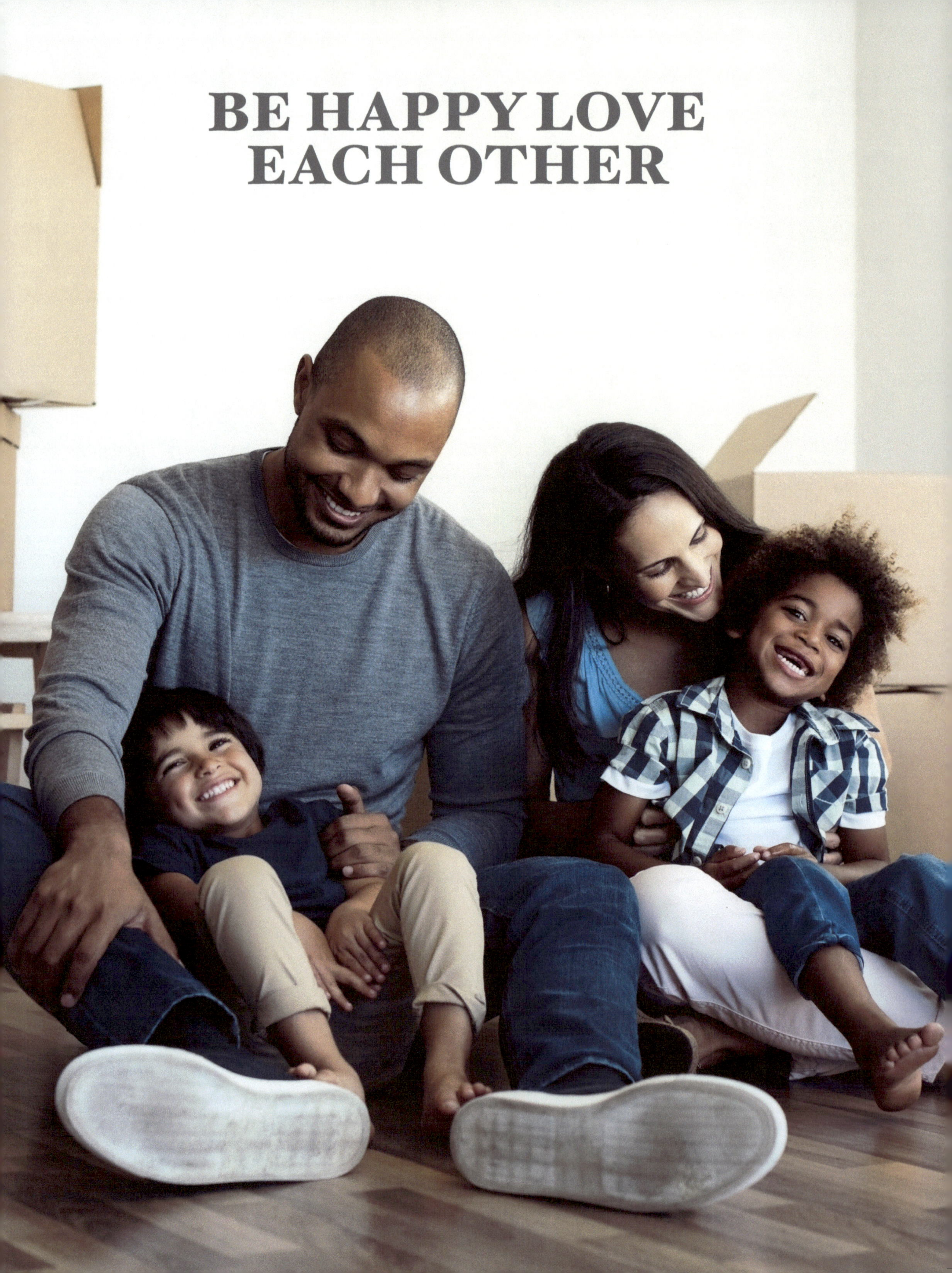
BE HAPPY LOVE
EACH OTHER

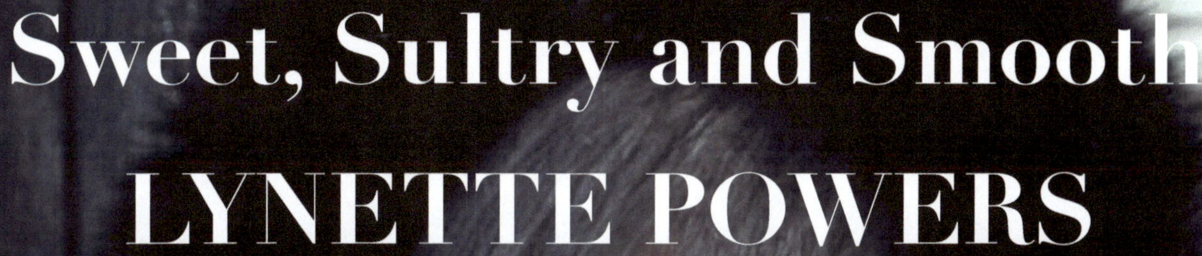

Sweet, Sultry and Smooth
LYNETTE POWERS

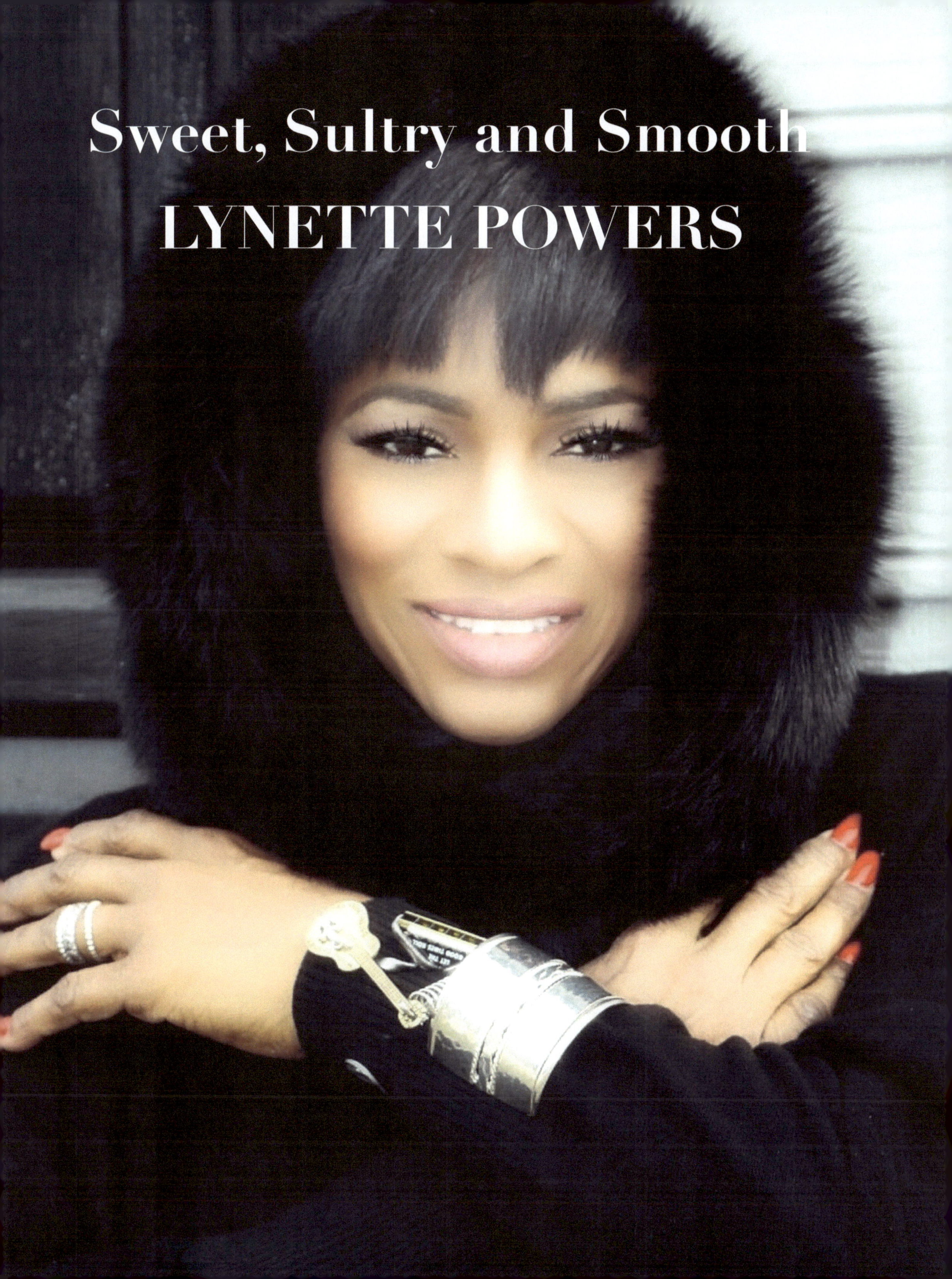

Sweet, Sultry and Smooth
LYNETTE POWERS

Lynette Powers uses her voice in various different styles, some of which we have not heard in a very long time. Lynette has the class of the late great Phyllis Hyman, the confidence and innocence of Ella Fitzgerald, and the sassiness of Sarah Vaughn with the brilliance and humbleness of Abby Lincoln. Her voice is magic, and it tells a story! Her passion has become her legacy because she is doing what she loves. A quote that Lynette lives by:

"I was born with music inside me. It was a force already with me when I arrived on the scene. It was a necessity for me like food to water." ~Ray Charles

Who is Lynette Powers?

Lynette Powers is a mother; wife; a daughter of music; a sister; a friend; a woman of faith and a musician who uses her creativity as a tool. It is a powerful tool of self-reflection, personal growth, survival and meant to inspire others to navigate the challenges and joys of life.

When did you know you wanted to sing?

As a child, I got my first taste of singing about age six in a small church in Camp Springs, Maryland. The first song I remember singing was called "Give Me My Flower While I Can Smell Them," with my two sisters LeAnn and LaVedia. As time went on, I performed in my junior high school glee club, the choir, countless open mic nights and with cover bands.

Are you from a musical family? Why jazz?

Yes. My parents William and Marion Powers were talented musicians. My dad played the percussions and my mother was a gifted vocalist who played the chitlin circuit with the Sunlight Stars in the 6Os. She also sang in the choir at 2nd Union Baptist Church in Washington, DC.

Jazz appeals to my love for all things abstract, especially art. I love all the possibilities and vibes that come with jazz. There are no limits on how I approach the music. I recall countless jam sessions with my parents, witnessing them engage in an amazing creative process. My dad and his friends would start with popular music of their time and transform it into something unique and remarkable, doing their own thing. Ultimately, I gravitate to a more organic sound, with an authentic vibe. I simply get a group of musicians and we start jamming.

Which famous vocalist do you admire most, and why?

That is a tough one for me because I love and admire so many artists, both men and women. They all have a special place in my soul and my life. But, if I must be specific, on a good day I channel my inner Billy Holiday, Phyllis Hyman, Al Jarreau and I love Jill Scott.

Sweet, Sultry and Smooth
LYNETTE POWERS

I love the texture of their voices, their expressions and the feeling underneath the songs they sing. They give me something to aspire to.

What inspires you to write?

Well, it is therapeutic for me. I look at the up and downs of my life, and all the in between. Music (my friend) saved me so many times. It is my go to. When I am alone, my music is my happy place. I can write about happy; I can write about sad; and I love to write love songs.

Singing has always carried me through the roller coaster ride my life has been at times. Good, bad or ugly, music got me through it. So, I write about stuff in the atmosphere.

What are your fondest musical memories?

Growing up back in the day, sitting on the stoop on Gault Place in NE Washington DC. It would be me and my girls Cynthia and Sharon Goodine, plus Terri West (Birdie) singing the Pointer Sisters' song "Jada's Coming Home." We sang our hearts out and the entire neighborhood was our audience. Those were the days! I also cherish the memories of gracing the stage in talent shows with Stacy Lattisaw and Johnny Gill. It was on and popping! I had the best time ever!

Is there a transformation when you hit the stage?

Well, I want to create a good energy, it is more than me just singing for me. I want the audience to vibe off me too! I truly feed off of their energy and spirit.

What inspired your new single and video "How Did We Get Here"?

It was a real relationship situation. I was going through something at the time and my niece (Teka) asked the question, how did we get here? She was going through something too. A concept was born. We commenced to writing about the crazy of it all. That line, "sitting beside you but you miles away," we all can relate to at some time or another. We all know that feeling of thinking, what is really going?

The year 2017 has been amazing to me! I've had the great fortune of working with a group of amazingly talented musicians and artists. As such, I have been challenged to grow as an individual and as a musician. From this process, new material was born! In 2018, you can look forward to the release of more new music from me. In the new year, I also plan to seek more opportunities to connect more with my audience, share more of myself and grow my fan base.

And there you have it! Ladies and gentlemen, Ms. Lynette Powers!

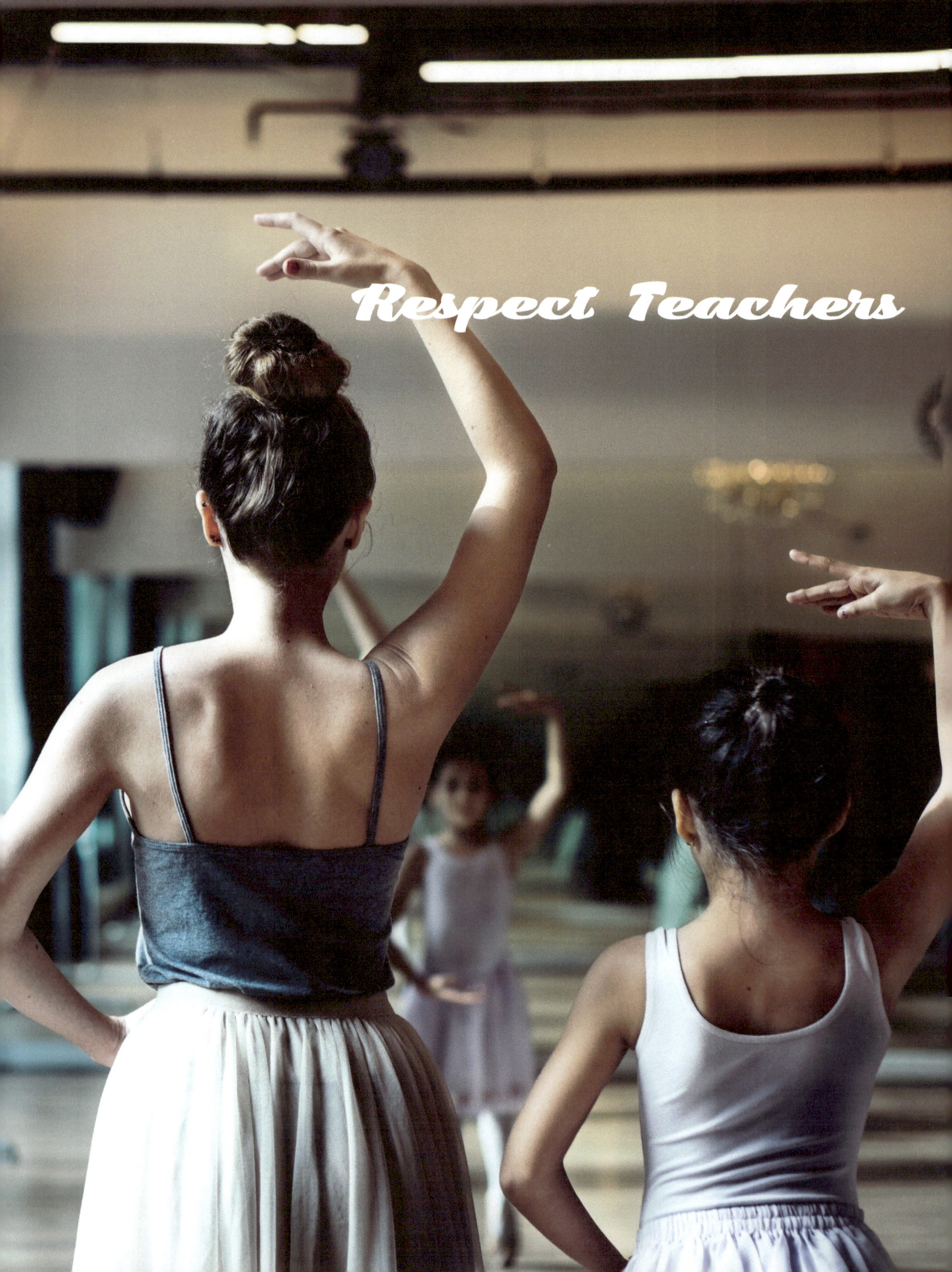
Respect Teachers

Welcome to 50 Round the Table, where the emphasis is on you "The Baby Boomer". This program is designed for people of a certain age and the particular situations they will experience. The challenges Baby Boomers have are many, but not as "uncommon" as most people would think. As we run our individual races in life, we all are focused on our independent finish line. However, there are situations that are, have and will be faced (head on) by us all at one time or another. We openly discuss issues of life as they pertain to our specific encounters. Topics that are discussed include, but are not limited to: physical fitness, mental fitness and nutritional values to further a greater quality of life.

Our discussions are open in nature. The 50 Round the Table forum will assist participants in furthering a more healthy, more vibrant and a more positive outlook of the rest of life. Some questions we ask are: "How do you want to love the rest of your life"? "Where do you fit in your life today"? "How do you want to live beneath your sky"?

We look forward to your comments, opinions and testimonials as we move to ward our greater selves.

Today's Subject is: "Bitterness vs Betterness"

"It is a simple but sometimes forgotten truth, that the greatest enemy to present joy and high hopes, is in the cultivation of retrospective bitterness" ~Robert G. Menzies

Bitterness in the now and in the future, stems from our not so welcomed past. When we look back on the negative, painful and sometimes regretful events that may have happened in our lives, and speak on them every chance we get, bitterness most times becomes our greatest ally. Whether it was never realizing a parental relationship with a father, a lover that did us wrong or even a missed opportunity caused by an unforeseen circumstance, bitterness has a peculiar technique of resurfacing when least expected. It is up to us to exorcise these demons and not allow them to consume our daily lives. We cannot allow these past events to invade, ruin and ultimately prevent us from moving forward.

"When the root is bitterness, imagine what the fruit might be…." ~Woodrow Kroll

We recognize a healthy tree by its strong, vascular root system. The most mature trees have roots that will break up sidewalks and damage foundations of homes when planted too closely. Bitterness has the same type of powerful roots, and is quickly recognized by the "fruit" (behavior) it bears. If you want the fruit of your life to be pleasant to the taste, we must rid ourselves of the need to hold onto the past and stretch toward the future with a greater expectation.

"Never succumb to the temptation of bitterness" ~Martin Luther King Jr.

One of our greatest leaders was met with opposition on every hand. He knew the situations he was facing had to change for the better. He knew the future generations were depending on him and his team to overcome the adversities of inequality. If he were to become bogged down in bitterness and accept "victim" to the oppression that was directly in his path, his children's children would never be able to thrive in the country of his birth. Bitterness had no place in his "tool box".

So now we look to be BETTER! It's the one and only state of being that will allow us the freedoms we deserve and should embrace. Good, better, best, never let it rest until our good is better and our better is our BEST! ~St. Jerome

We must understand that when we give way to the better things, ideas and behaviors, the Law of Attraction also shifts. Many have read literature that contains such sayings as; "What you sow you will reap", "What goes around comes around", "Do unto others as you would have them do unto you", etc…. We recognize these verses and often times use them to our advantage. But when the rubber meets the road, so to speak, we have the tendency to lash out, and revert to what we embrace negative reaction.

Forgiveness is a huge part of BETTERNESS. I've heard it said, that the act of forgiving my fellow man should be as urgent and important as the quickness with which I'd like God to forgive me. To err is human, but to forgive is divine. It is time to move forward, time to let go of the grudges we may have been holding against those with which we've been given command to peacefully coexist. The amusing thing about grudges, is that much of the ought we may have against our fellow man is not ours to harbor. It has been given to us through gossip and conversation.

When we run toward bettering ourselves, there will be opposition. Misery does love company and they are not going to be willing to set you free. Stay on course. Utilize motivational speakers, motivational books and keep your eyes forward. The windshield is much bigger than the rearview mirror for a reason. The only thing you should back in to is a parking space.

Your future is waiting for you to arrive. Be whole and fully intact, discovering all the world as your playground. Frolic and rejoice in YOUR new beginning. Be your authentic self, be your best self. There is no room for bitterness in your life….ONLY BETTERNESS!

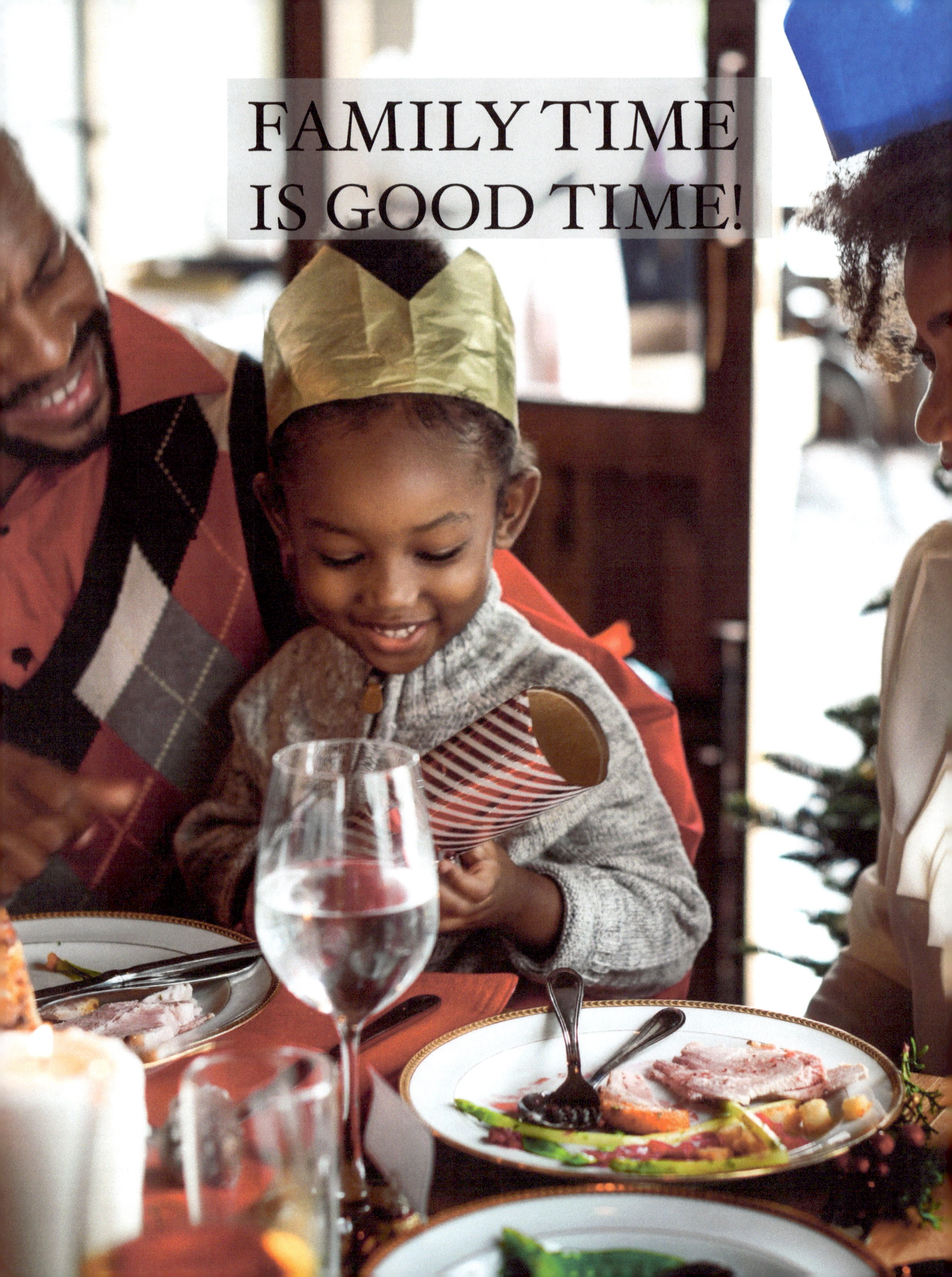

FAMILY TIME
IS GOOD TIME!

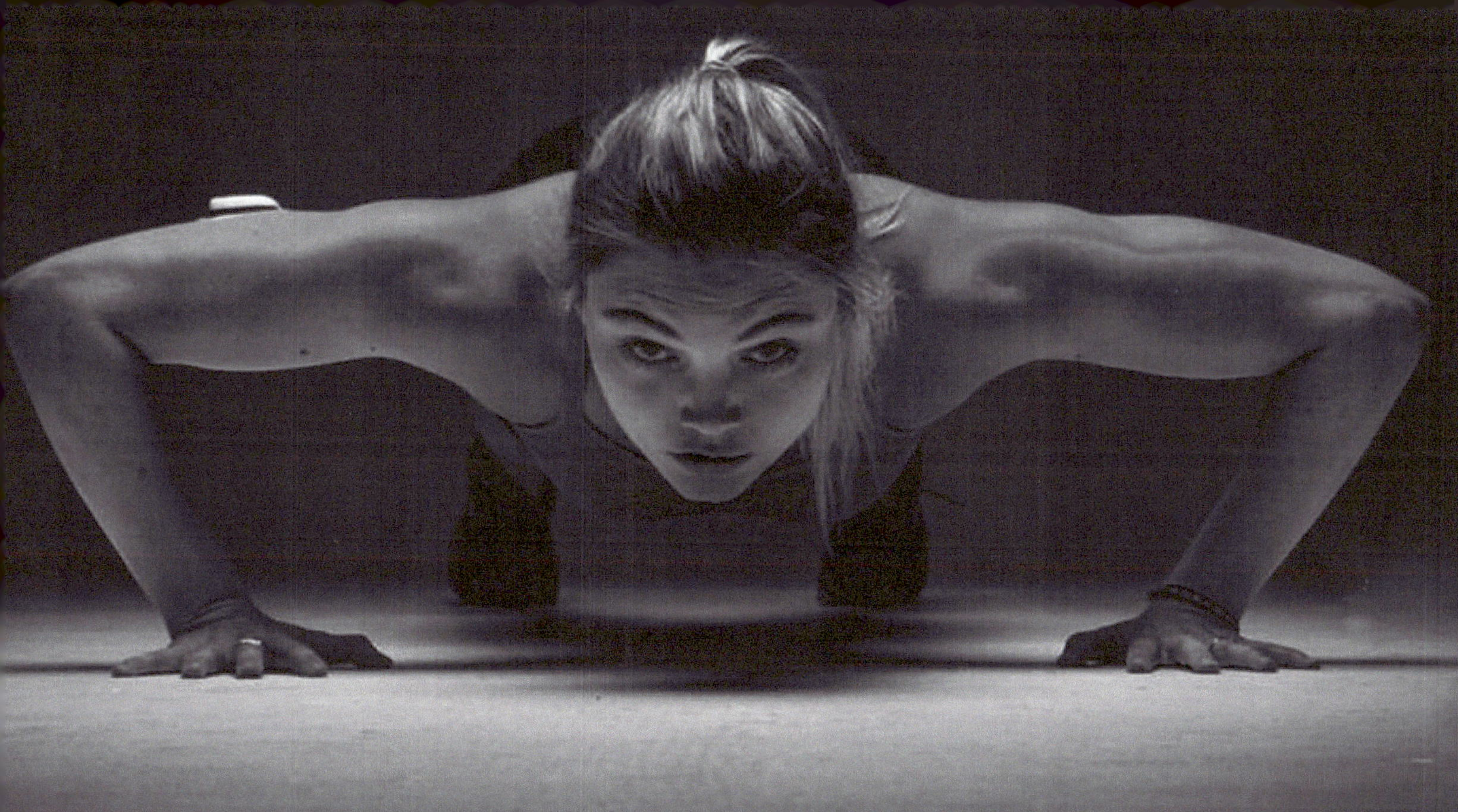

BECAUSE SHE NEVER GAVE UP

Good afternoon Alex, you have a very motivating story of staying positive while dealing with type one Diabetes. Tell our readers a little about why you didn't give up.

Well, I'm an Atlanta native, born in Fulton County. I grew up, attended high school, college, and even met and married my husband, whom is also named Alex. As a child, I always had a passion for dance and my own unique style. I took dance classes from the age of 2 until I graduated from high school. Always an active child I competed in various sports. Even after the diagnosis of type one diabetes at the age of 13.

What were your thoughts when you knew Diabetes wasn't something that was easy to live with?

Sports enabled me to begin learning that perseverance was more important than just talent. I tore my ACL in high school and had to work hard to come back to sports and dance. This gave me an appreciation for hard work and drive by demonstrating how overcoming could be a reward on its own. Modeling had always been a dream of mine, as I loved watching Americas Next Top Model with my younger sister. In the spring of 2014, GOD handed me an amazing opportunity to reach my dream. However, it would not come without hard work and perseverance. I filled out an entry for a talent search in the local mall, competed, and won. The best part was that it included a trip to New York City. However, before I could take my trip I was hospitalized for the third time with Diabetic Ketoacidosis (DKA) which is a complication from diabetes that can be serious and life-threatening. It occurs when there is not enough insulin in the body to break down glucose and ketones are released. Therefore, the body turns to breaking down fat as fuel, but after it runs out of fat, it begins to target muscles and organs. The reason I didn't have enough insulin in my body was because I wasn't taking any insulin in attempts to lose weight. I had struggled with eating disorders and body dysphoria for many years, even before my diabetes diagnosis. I attempted to manipulate my weight in other unhealthy ways as well.

BECAUSE SHE NEVER GAVE UP

About 2 weeks after I returned home from the hospital, I had a photo shoot with my scouts. I did not want to inform them of my recent hospitalization, but I had gained 15-20 pounds after using insulin, I didn't have much of a choice. In that moment, I expected to lose it all, to have the dream yanked out of my grasp. However, rather than being critical, they were supportive. They encouraged me to get to the gym and get healthy. They didn't take my trip away; they simply put it on hold until I was ready to go physically and mentally. That day, my mom and I joined the gym together, and I began working hard to be healthy and strong.

Why do you feel that modeling makes you so happy?

I feel like modeling saved my life! Having my dreams on the line caused me to fight to be healthy. It was, and continues to be a fight, but I persevere knowing that anything worth doing takes hard work and determination. My work has paid off, and God continues to provide me awesome opportunities, including runway shows in Atlanta, New York, Memphis and Huntsville; and walking for amazing designers such as Van Miller International. My print work can be seen in Modern Luxury Brides, Impact Atlanta Fashion & Beauty , Southern Living Magazine, and Gainesville Times Brides; Brand Ambassador work for Beauty Water, Kellelogs, Resespeezes, and Urban Scholar; hair shows for multiple salons and brands such as Van Michael Salon, The David K. Space, Salon Red, Bigen, Indique, and Taliah Waajid; and social media commercials for fitness facilities. I've twice been nominated for Atlanta's Hottest Model and won in 2017. In addition to my modeling work I have worked as an extra for an upcoming film, and was casted in "Damnation," a stage play by Russel Tyson.

Where do you see yourself in the future?

As I look to the future, I want to continue to use my modeling as a platform to raise awareness for type 1 diabetes and eating disorders, and also to encourage others in knowing that no matter what obstacles they may face to chase their dreams. Long term I also hope to open an outpatient rehabilitation center for those struggling with eating disorders.

What would be your advice to other models?

My advice to those looking to get in to the industry is don't be afraid of hard work or rejection. Just because you are not picked for something does not mean there is anything wrong with you. Find your market and capitalize on it! Also, remember to stay thankful and humble, surround yourself with positive and supportive people. You may have rough times, hell, you will have rough times, but that's okay, just pick yourself back up and carry on. Just don't lose yourself in the process. Always remember, "All things are possible through Christ who strengthens me." Philippians 4:13 Some of Alex's work can be seen on the next six pages. A true story of perseverance and never giving up!

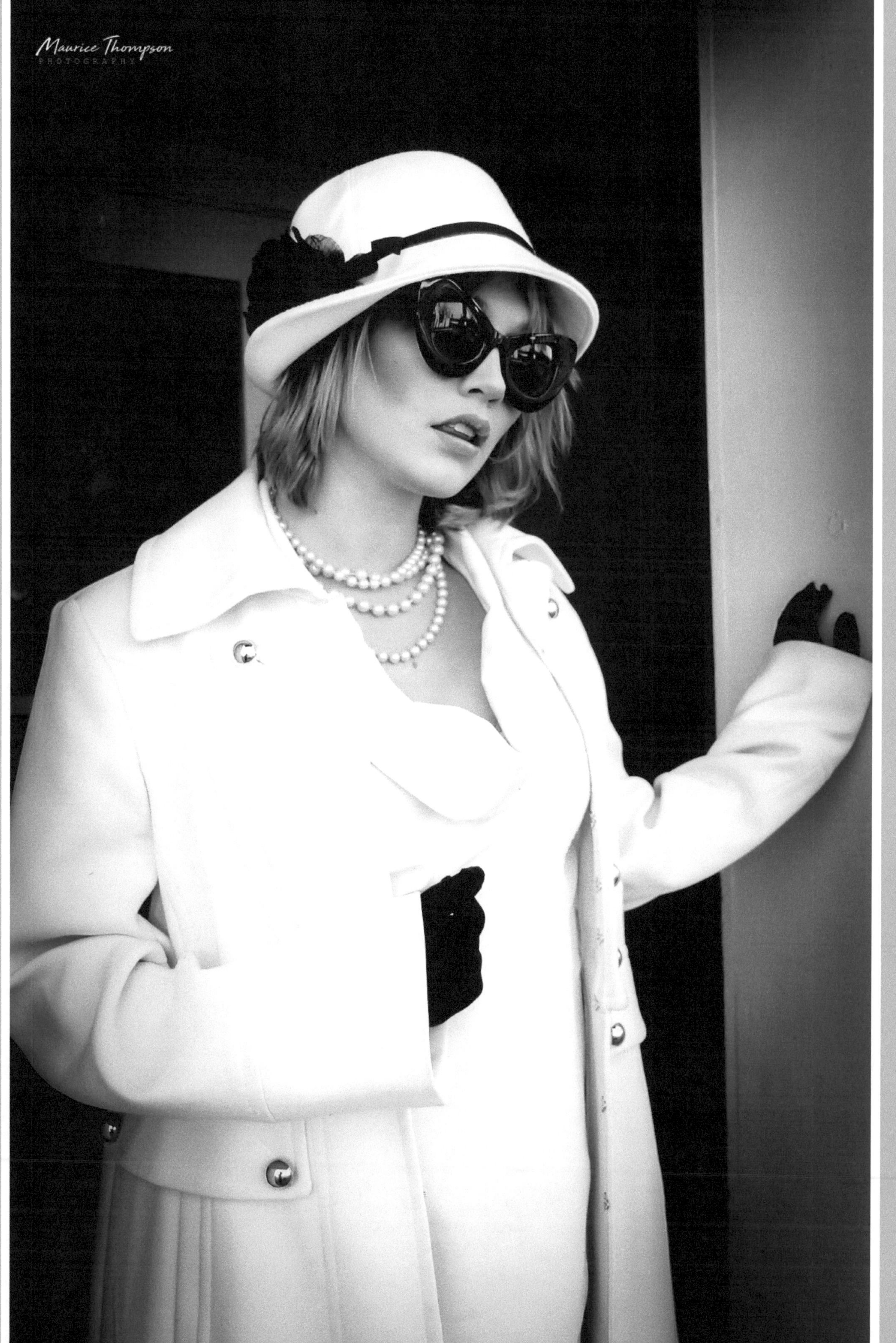
Maurice Thompson
PHOTOGRAPHY

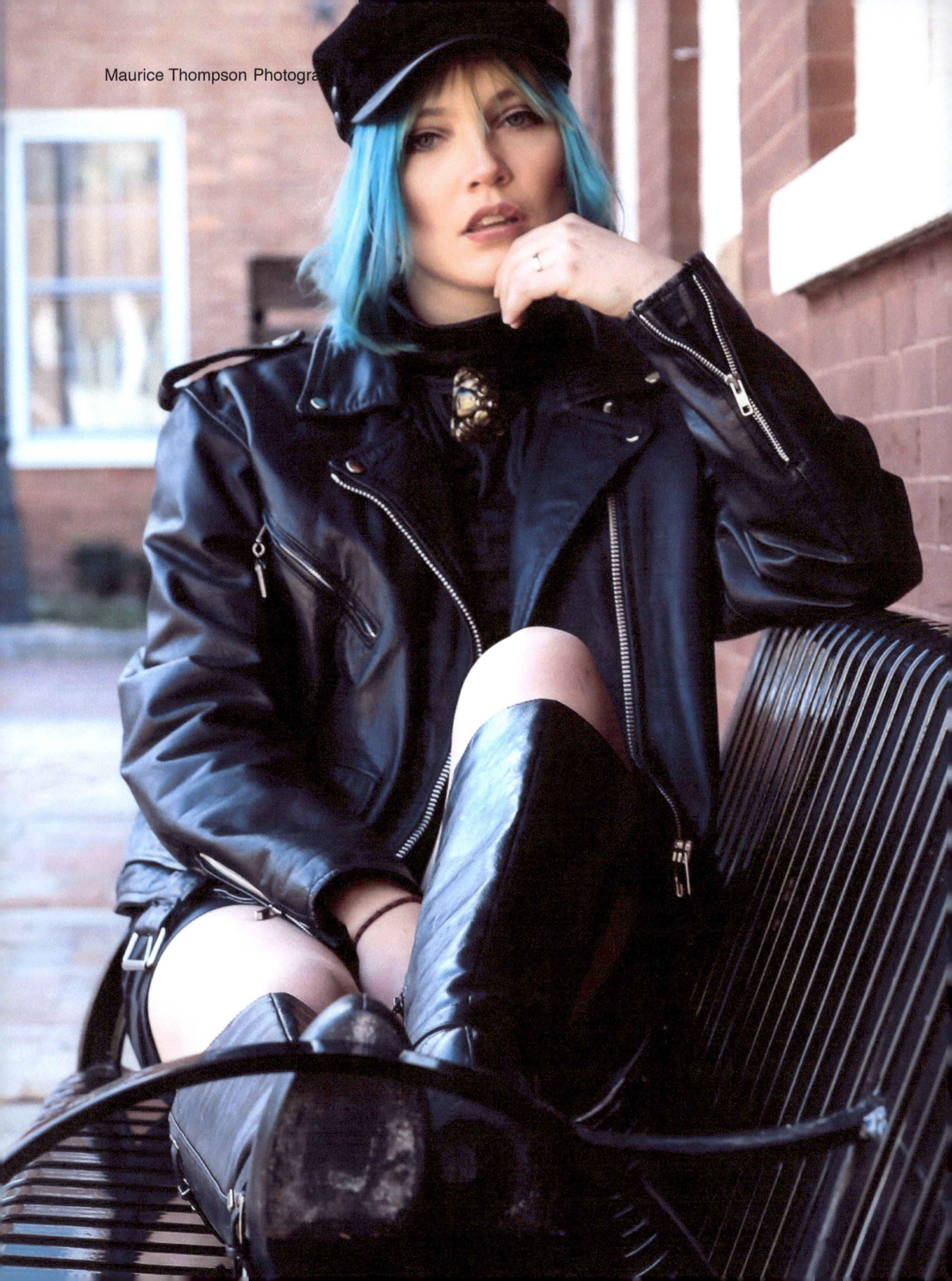
Maurice Thompson Photogra

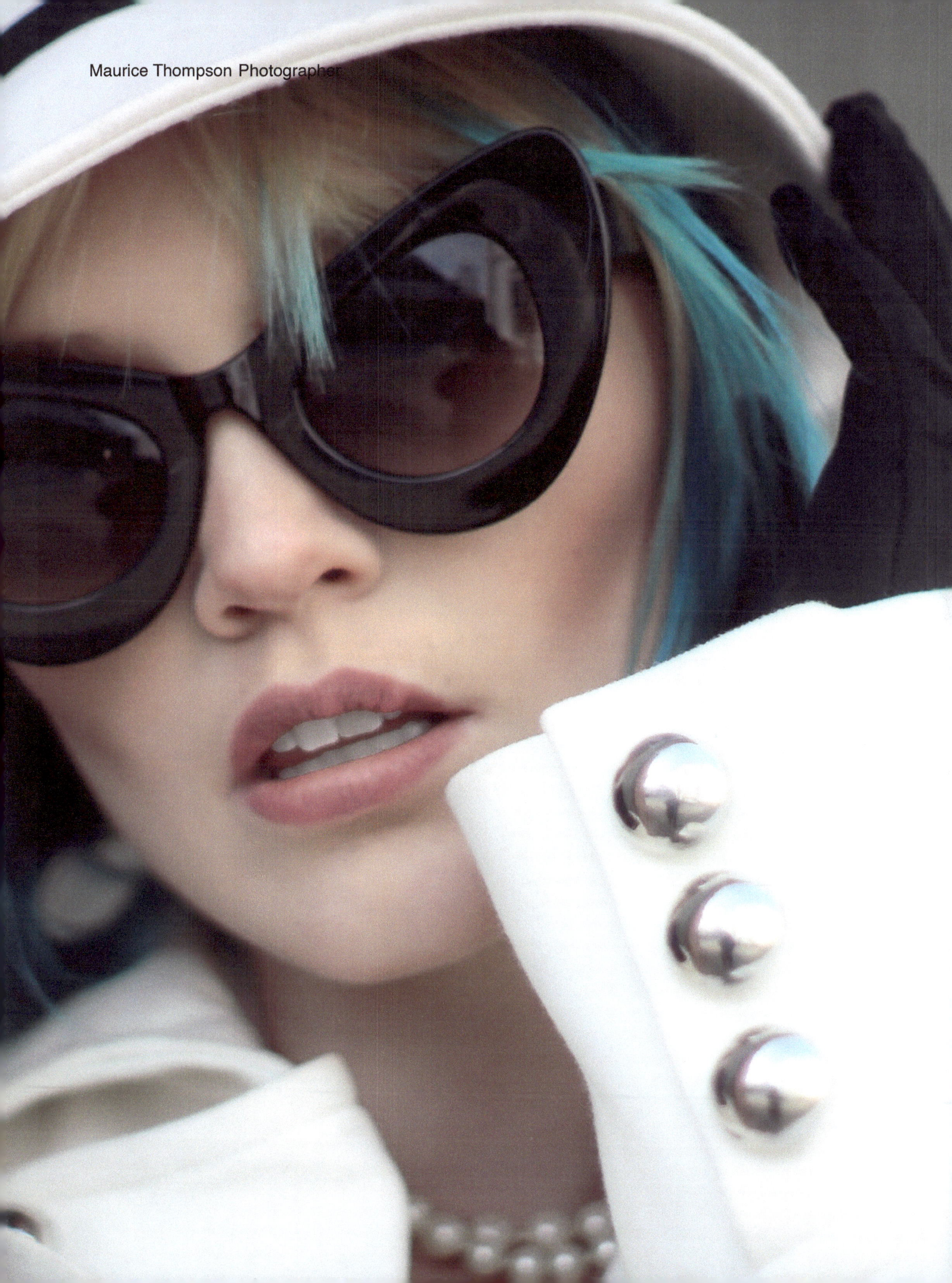
Maurice Thompson Photographer

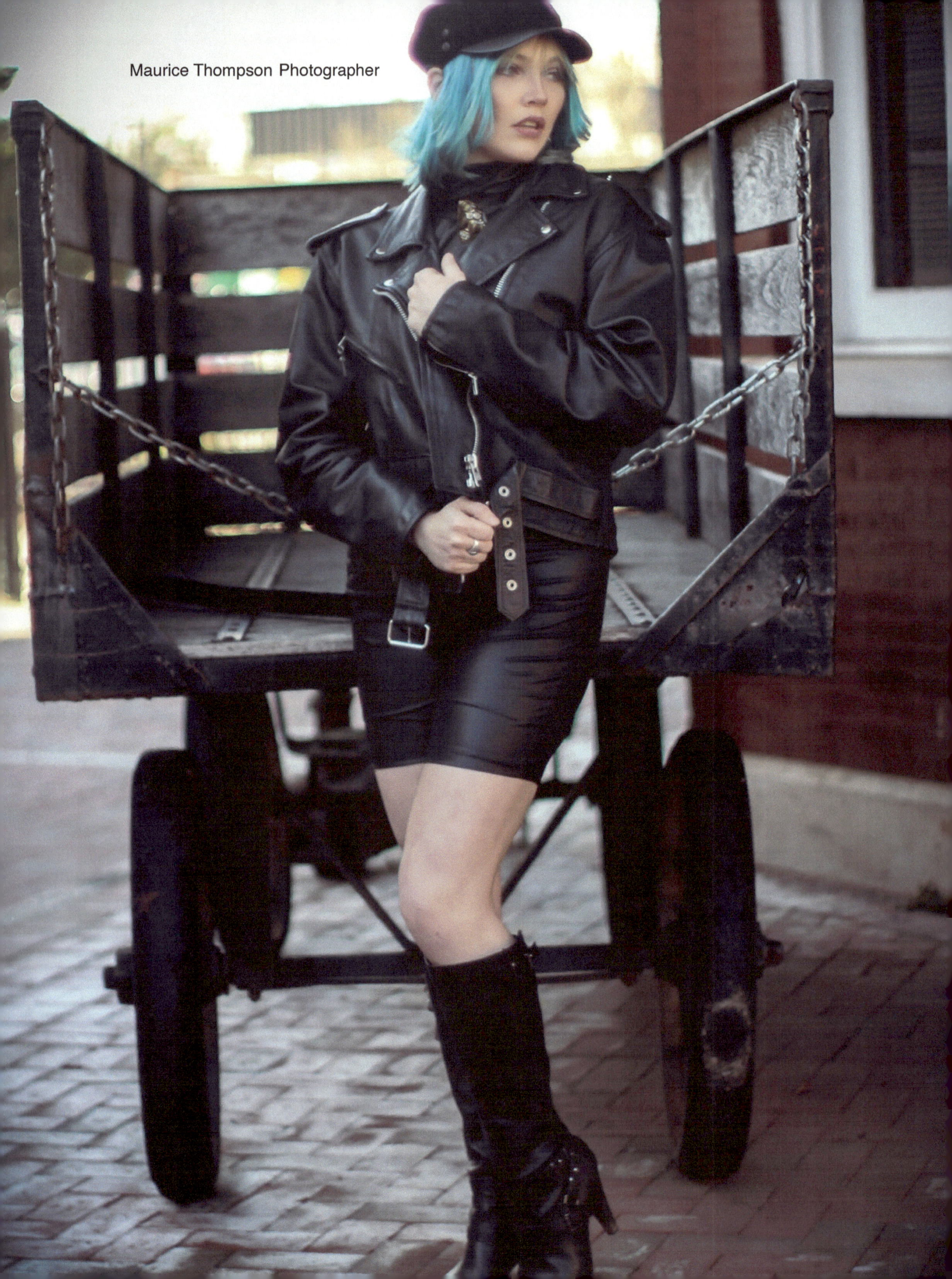
Maurice Thompson Photographer

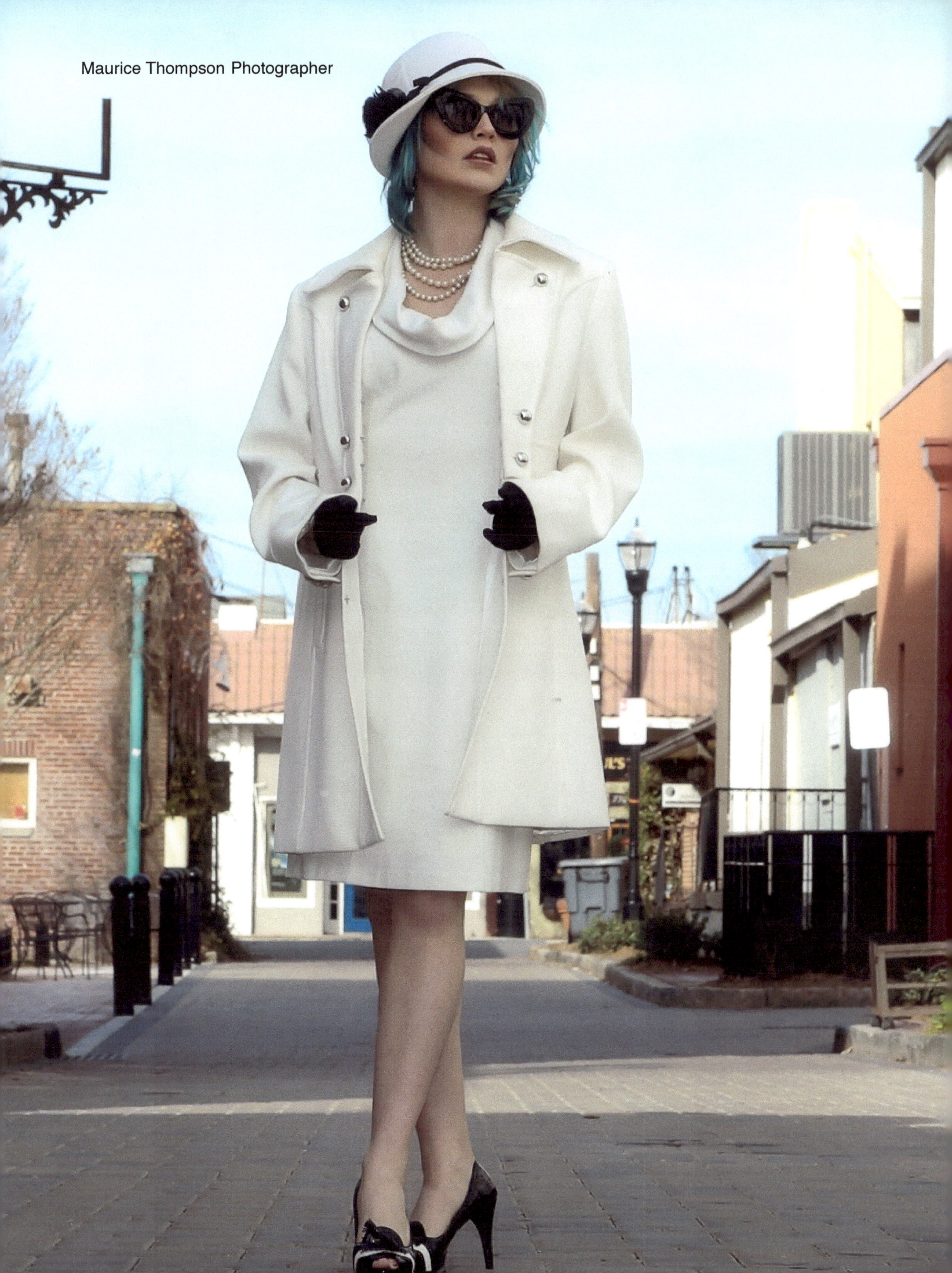
Maurice Thompson Photographer

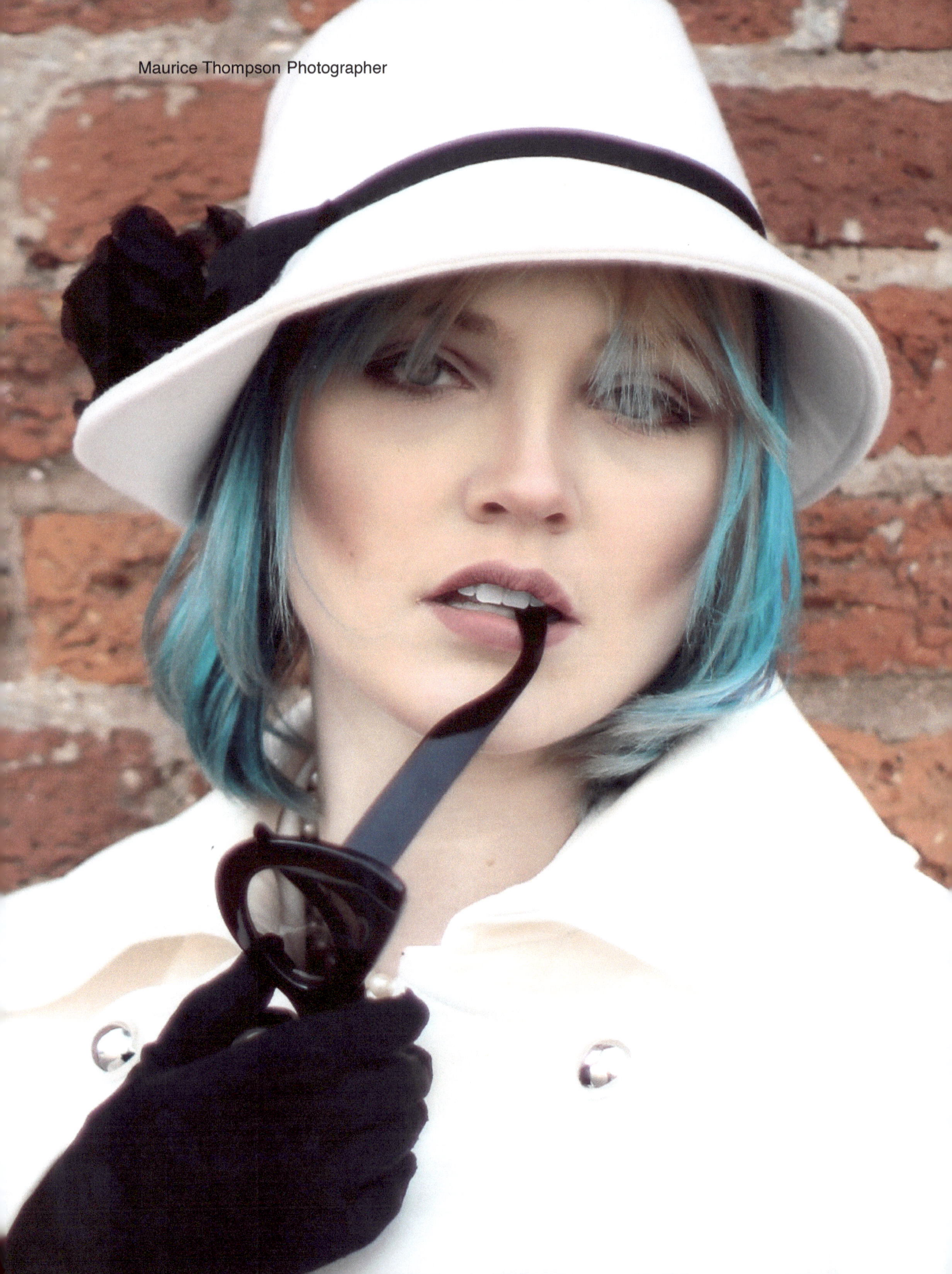
Maurice Thompson Photographer

DEXTER TUCKER
HOME, FAMILY, CAREER AND THE BLESSINGS

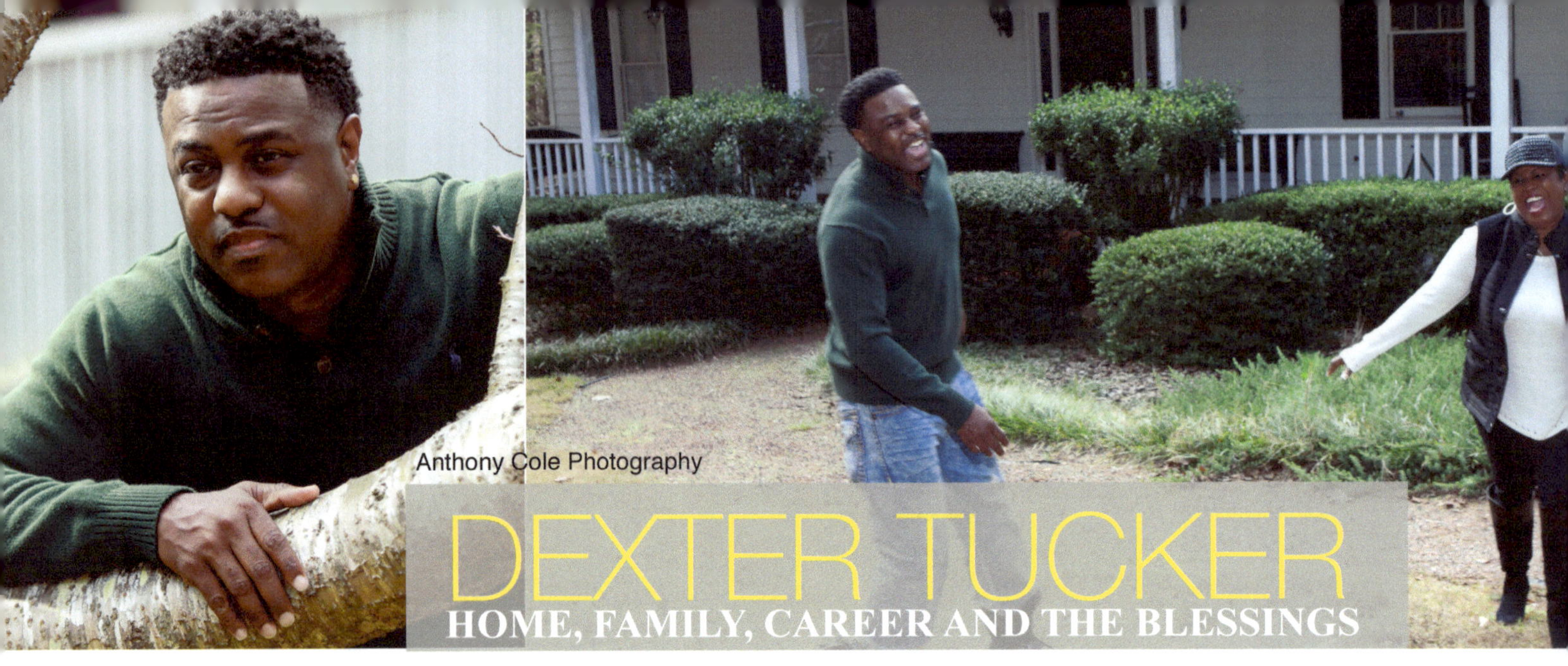

DEXTER TUCKER
HOME, FAMILY, CAREER AND THE BLESSINGS

As I look around I feel the love of home, family, career and the blessings. I also had the opportunity to chat briefly with his backbone, Dexters beautiful wife Jo. Thank you Jo for such a warm welcome into your home on this early Saturday morning. As we sip tea, Dexter comes out and joins us. What an honor it is to have this candid opportunity to learn more about one of the hardest working men in the entertainment business.

IAM: Dexter, you are Atlanta born and raised; you have toured all over the United States doing stand-up comedy, appeared in movies, stage plays, even hosted various events over the past fifteen years. You also co-hosted the *Nollywood Films* Critics' awards (*NAFCA*) *African Oscars*, alongside Omarosa Manigualt, in Hollywood California. Most recently now a filmmaker with several notable projects under your belt.

You are the older brother of the famed funny man Chris Tucker. Most people are familiar with Chris Tucker, tell our readers about Dexter Tucker?

DEXTER: Dexter is a little black boy from the East side of Atlanta growing up in Decatur my entire life, raised Christian by my mom and born December 12th., which makes me a Sagittarius. I read my horoscope this morning and it said something like I'm the type of person that has a lot going on at one time, sort of a jack of all trades, master of none type of guy. But as I have gotten older I started to recognize and define things about myself. Even though I'm pretty good at everything I do, I master nothing. So yeah that's me! So, after reading my horoscope I told myself I could not live like that. I have goals, so I'll take on new projects in a minute. Even though I feel like I'm about twenty five, people must remind me of how old I really am. In fact the only thing that makes me feel older is watching my girls get older.

IAM: How many girls do you have?

DEXTER: I have three girls ages, twenty five, eighteen and sixteen.

IAM: What I have observed outside of your career you are a family man, spending a lot of time with your wife and children. You are known for inviting old school friends to your home for pool parties or to just hang out. Dexter, what does home mean to you?

DEXTER: I think I got that from my dad. When we were young we would BBQ (that's what we call cookouts here in the South). Often the whole neighborhood would show up, to include my entire family. By the way I come from a large family. All very funny, especially my dad, who is the real comedian.

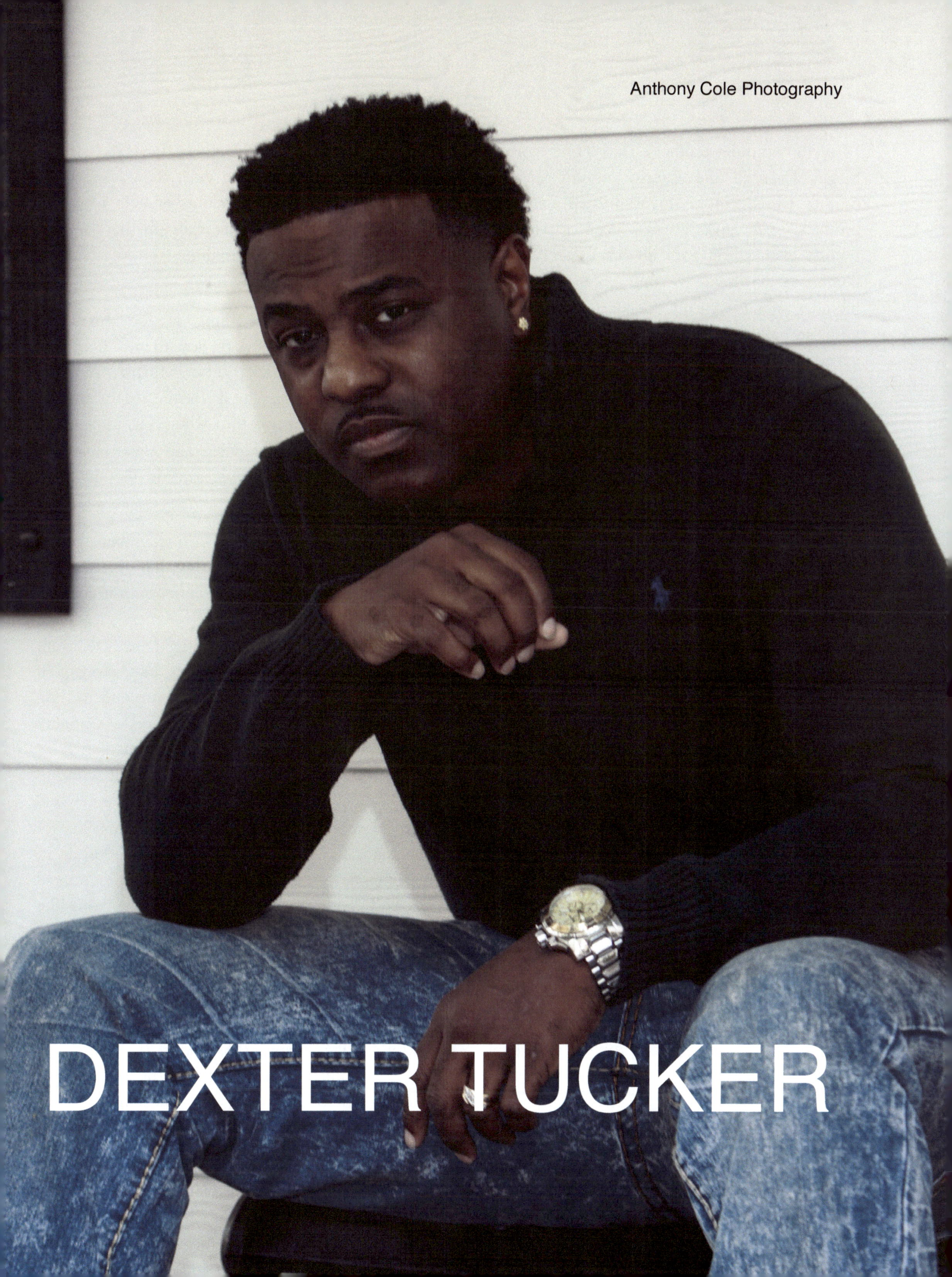

Anthony Cole Photography
DEXTER TUCKER

I have a two older brothers, Darryl and Norris Jr. Sisters Lucretia and Tammy, myself and baby brother Chris. Not to mention step sisters and brothers. We have always been a close-knit family, even Chris with all his fame. We were taught to be loyal to one another, and that includes friends. All my friends I went to school with are all still friends to this day. I prefer spending time with them because I know their friendship and their love is unconditional for me. So, to sum it up Home is unconditional.

IAM: What is the biggest misconception that people may have of you?

DEXTER: I would say the fact that people thought that I was just pursuing a career in comedy because my brother is big in the industry. The funny thing is, I always knew in the forefront of my mind that everyone was going to say that. I knew the comedy game was no joke. I wanted to be good and Chris being my brother was not going to help me be good. Look, people will boo you right off the stage. Trust me people would love to boo me just because I'm Chris Tucker's brother. Another thing I would hear people saying is, "He don't like people to say he is Chris Tuckers brother," and that's just not true. Chris is my brother first unconditionally, then he is Chris Tucker the mega star. He is my brother and I couldn't be prouder to be his big brother. Besides, I'm on my grind trying hard to be funny and build my own brand. I also knew it would take time, but let's be very clear about this one thing, I have never envied my brother, his success, or career.

IAM: So, you never had a problem with people saying that you are living in your brother's shadow?

DEXTER: No, I know more about this game than people give me credit for, honestly. I have been around it for many years and I took the same route as all other comedians. I have done open mics, hole in the walls, ran the chitiln circuits,

Sunday boo nights. Basically, I did it all. And if people don't do anything else, they respect me because I did not get handouts or help from my brother. I have earned my spot on the comedic stage. I never expected anything from my brother, nor did I ever ask for anything.

IAM: What do you think is the difference between the comedians on top then and now, I mean then we had Eddie Murphy, Martin Lawrence, the late great Bernie Mac and of course Chris Tucker. All of whom has gone on to do great things in movies, and now have big careers. Who do we have now on that level of funniness beside yourself?

DEXTER: We have plenty of that caliber, but the difference is the fact that during that time the late 80s early and mid-90s it was a hot era for comics. Take rap for instance, when it was first introduced to America it was something new. Def Jam introduced comedy as something new and mixed it with HIP HOP! That made everyone excited about comedy. So, when you turn on Def Comedy Jam you saw "US," young black comedians. We could curse, get wild with it, and mix it with hip hop collaborated with the likes of Kid Capri. Man that was a special time, and after that it got oversaturated because everybody wanted to do it. Then came Comic View on BET. They let almost anybody get on stage. DEF Comedy Jam was like a tight fraternity and a lot of those guys ended up being great superstars and rightfully so.

IAM: You have appeared in movies like *Money Talk with Chris Tucker*, *My Big Fat Hip Hop Family*, *Lynch Mob*, *Treasure in the Hood* and most recently you were very instrumental in two movies where not only did you have starring roles, you also had the opportunity to co-write, produce and direct these films. *One, The Comedy Club Movie,* and the other *Jimmy Part 1 (did you get one)* both slated for a spring release. Dexter what motivates your versatility.

DEXTER: When I made the decision to get into comedy it was not to just be a comedian but to get in the business of "show business." Do not misunderstand me, I love being a comic. It is very challenging and rewarding. I love to make people laugh. But I can honestly say that at this point in my life I'm more interested in the production side of the business, with an acting role here and there. Of course I will forever be funny, now that will never change it's in the bloodline. Because I got a late start in this game it's now what I like to call chess not checkers. Every move is strategic.

IAM: What do you take the most pride in? Where is your passion?

DEXTER: My passion right now is being a great filmmaker. I think my biggest accomplishment is finishing a movie, and it was hard to get people on the same page with very little budget.

IAM: I get it! In fact, it's a rare find when you do find a group of people willing to work for very little or pro bono and hang in until the end. Let's talk about Dexter the filmmaker, how did that begin?

DEXTER: Well at one time I thought becoming a filmmaker would be easy, in fact my first film was shot with my partners at that time Rick Stephenson and Derrick Handspike with XtraPoint films. We all came together to do a movie written and created by Rick Stephenson. I came in as co-writer, producer and creative director. The movie is called, *The Comedy Club Movie*. The goal with the movie was to create an outlet for comedians in the community to have a place for their talent, a platform for exposure. The concept was for it to take off like a *Friday* movie in Atlanta, and at the very least we would have an opportunity to work.

IAM: Can you tell our readers about the plot of the *Comedy Club* movie?

DEXTER: Well the premise of the movie is very simple. It is about a few guys that are friends and trying to start a comedy night at a night club. Something I have done in my real life. But these are just some regular guys working nine to five, and one of them had a great desire to be a promoter. Plus he thought his friends were funny. So he got on a mission to start a comedy night at a club. The movie follows him on this mission and all the adversity and stumbling blocks that he ran into trying to make it work. It took some time to shoot the movie with all the ups and downs, but with determination we finished the movie and now looking for a spring release.

IAM: I understand that the movie got rave reviews in the Poconos Film Festival. In fact the movie was nominated in the independent film category as best comedy by the NAFCA Nollywood Film Critics' Awards, as well as a nomination for Ms. Chrystale Wilson best supporting actress in a comedy. That is a great accomplishment and certainly something to be proud of.

DEXTER: After the completion of the movie Derrick Handspike and I shopped the movie in New York and LA seeking distribution. Because this was all new to the both of us we realize we had to work harder to overcome the obstacle to be competitive in the industry. I mentioned earlier that they really do not care how funny you are, what matters is how many ticket can you sell; whether it is on stage or at the movie theater. We are now to the point where the movie can be released, so that is exciting.

IAM: So, I understand that you ventured into a second film project?

DEXTER: Exactly! My partner Jerry May, another young inspiring filmmaker, approached me with a concept he had about a horror suspense movie. Jerry and I collaborated on my second movie called, *Jimmy Part I (Did you get one)*. I have the lead role in the film, and Joelena Tucker plays my wife.

IAM: Yes, I had the opportunity to attend the premier of the movie awesome job!

DEXTER: Thank you! I'm very proud of that movie because it was self-funded. Jerry and I own the Movie and it is set up for a sequel.

IAM: Smart move, I want to ask you about the blessing! What can we look forward to from Dexter Tucker in 2018?

DEXTER: Wow the blessing is everything that I have spoke about here today. It's a blessing that I have two projects that will be released in 2018 that will solidify me as a filmmaker. I'm looking forward to greater exposure of my filmmaking talents here in Atlanta, alongside Tyler Perry and Will Packer. In 2017 Atlanta became number one in film in the world. It has been a great motivating factor for me to complete projects and not just have shelf ideas. So, the blessing is that scripts are now complete, and budgets are coming together. I have learned a lot about how important it is to have quality movies, and how important it is to have a budget for marketing/promotion and distribution. I'm also co-starring in a movie alongside DMX called *Doggman,* which we will begin shooting early 2018. Prayerfully we can look for a summer release as I simultaneously compete for a Netflix standup comedy special, as well as the release of the *Andre Rison Life Story*. Which I might add is a very interesting story outside of what the public knows of him and Lisa (Left Eye) Lopez (R.I.P.). We introduce and shed light on Andre the man, his history in the NFL and his involvement in the entertainment industry. So, I have some really big things happening for 2018 with Off Glenwood Entertainment, my partner Deondai Colquitt, from Xtrapoint Films Rick Stephenson and Derrick Handspike; as well as Jerry May of Jerry May Production. I also cannot forget my awesome attorney, Kendall Minter. They are the people I work very closely with, and that is a blessing! The things I have learned I have instilled into my children. If you figure out what you want to do early in life and stay persistent you can achieve anything. Like a drop of water dripping on a rock eventually that dripping water will drip a hole in that rock if it drips long enough. Then you will see true success. What people cannot take away for from you is experience. I am at a point in my life where I have had some success, and I like the way it taste. Now I am hungry for more. I will always do comedy, and believe me I have a lot to say, I'm a father, I'm a husband and I'm a hustler. I am never going to get on a stage and crack jokes, I'm always going to talk about real life. I'm more focused now then ever before. This Sagittarius is now a jack of all trade and a master of something. Now that's what I call being blessed!

IAM: Sounds like 2018 is going to be a golden year for you. Dexter It's been a pleasure Chatting with you. Thanks so much.

Among the Lavender Fields

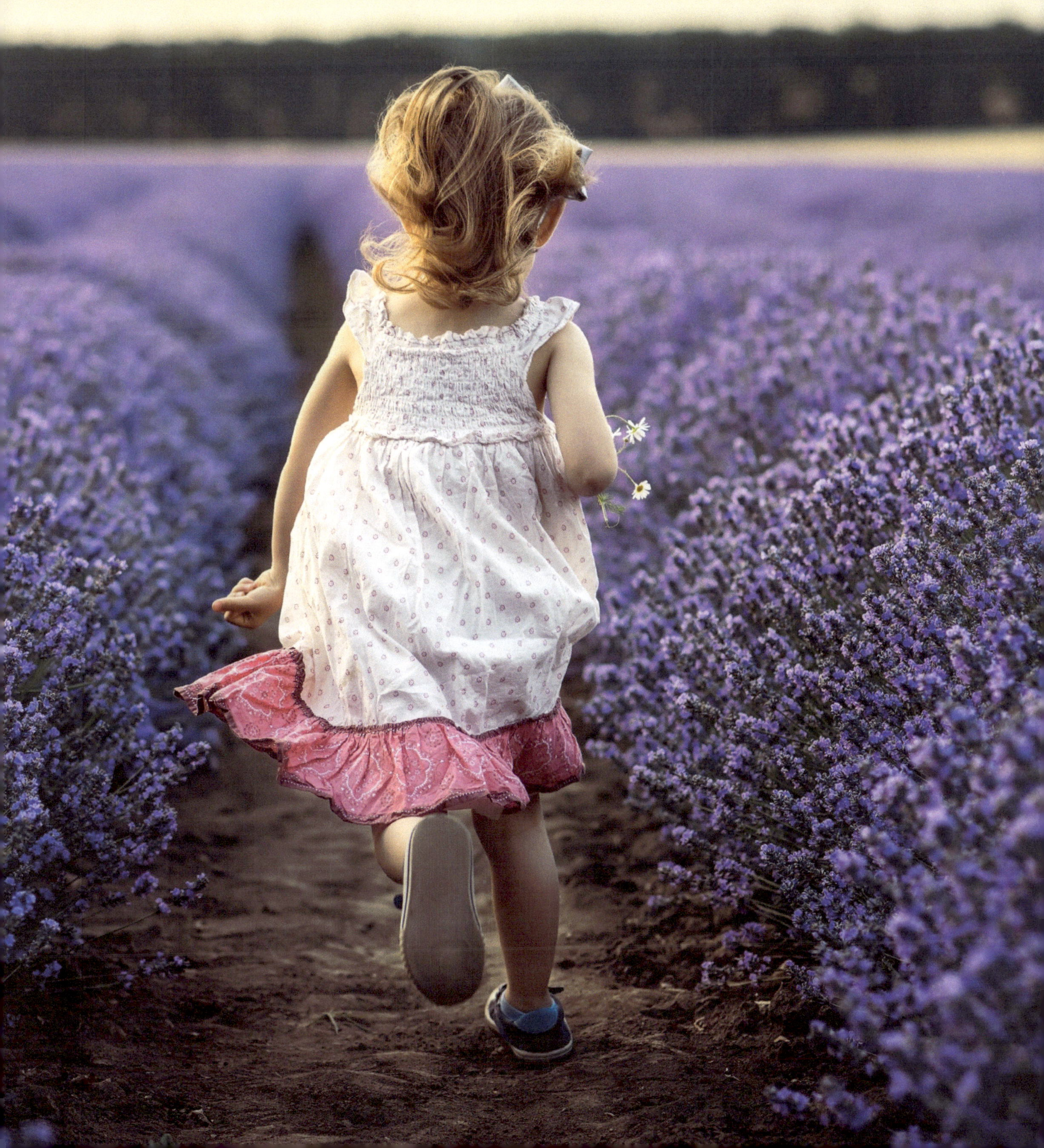

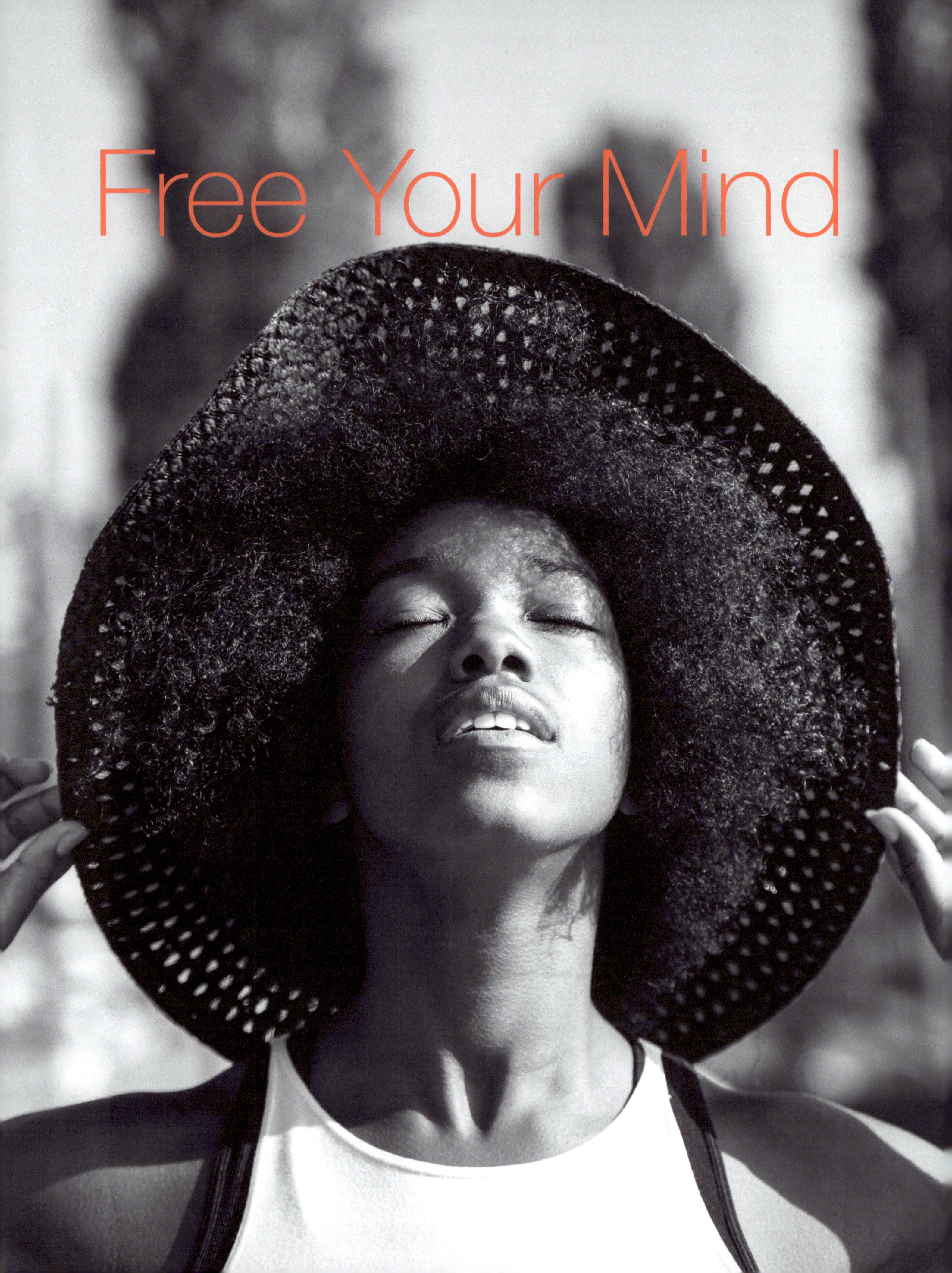
Free Your Mind

www.ingramcontent.com/pod-product-compliance
Lightning Source LLC
Chambersburg PA
CBHW040200240726
48664CB00002B/778